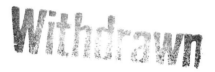

HEALING YOUR HUNGRY HEART

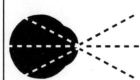 This Large Print Book carries the
Seal of Approval of N.A.V.H.

HEALING YOUR HUNGRY HEART

RECOVERING FROM YOUR EATING DISORDER

JOANNA POPPINK, MFT

THORNDIKE PRESS
A part of Gale, Cengage Learning

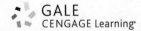

GALE
CENGAGE Learning·

Detroit • New York • San Francisco • New Haven, Conn • Waterville, Maine • London

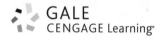
GALE
CENGAGE Learning®

LIBRARY OF CONGRESS CATALOGING-IN-PUBLICATION DATA

Poppink, Joanna.
    Healing your hungry heart : recovering from your eating disorder / Joanna Poppink.
        p. cm.---(Thorndike Large print health, home,& learning)
        ISBN 978-1-4104-4441-7 (hardcover : large print) — ISBN 1-4104-4441-4 (hardcover : large print) 1. Eating disorders. 2. Eating disorders—Treatment. 3. Large type books. I. Title.
    RC552.E18P67 2012
    616.85'26—dc23   2011041222

Published in 2012 by arrangement with Conari Press, an imprint of Red Wheel/Weiser, LLC.

Printed in the United States of America
1 2 3 4 5 6 7 16 15 14 13 12

CONTENTS

ACKNOWLEDGMENTS

Thank you to my editors, Amber Guetebier and Sandy Doell, for your support, life experience, caring, and expertise; Kevin Bellows, friend and editor; Jeanne Rust, for listening to my struggles and being a constant source of love and support.

Thank you Jennifer Armstrong, my technology guru, who freed me from communication complexities by simplifying my computer processing.

Thank you members of IWOSC (Independent Writers of Southern California), particularly Alice Romano and Melanie Chartoff and the UCLA Writers Program for sharing your expertise and encouragement.

Thank you to every patient I've ever worked with for your courage, wisdom, and trust as you shared your journey to recovery with me.

Thank you to my great friends and teachers — especially Lars and Ingeborg Lofgren and Hedda Bolgar — for your words of wisdom ringing and whispering in my mind. Your guidance in my own recovery path was always mixed with love.

Thank you to my daughter, Deborah, and my son-in-law, David, for your steadfast confidence that I would succeed. And thanks to my terrier, Winston, who is always ready to take a walk when I need a break from writing.

Most of all, I acknowledge and am grateful to my two granddaughters who, at the time of this writing, are three and five years old; Hannah Jane Rainbow and Delilah Noel Starfish. You continually gave me your uninhibited love, support, and inspiration — plus encouraging art work. You inspired me and provided constant examples of the healthy, creative, and joyous feminine life spirit that needs to be fostered, cherished, and respected by us all.

Dedicated to the spirit of life, joy,
and wisdom in all women.

AUTHOR'S NOTE

The perspective and suggestions shared in this book are not a substitute for medical advice. If you think you have an eating disorder, please contact your doctor or another qualified healthcare professional very soon to discuss the emotions and behaviors that trouble you.

CHAPTER 1
UNREAL TO REAL:
SNAPSHOTS OF MY STORY

"Self-observation is an instrument of
self-change, a means of awakening."
— George Gurdjieff

I started making myself throw up when I
was thirteen years old and didn't stop for
thirty years. I hope that the snapshots of my
story and other women's stories in this
book, coupled with my own healing and
recovery work with women for over twenty-
five years, can help you find your personal
path to recovery. Within the pages of these
shared experiences, please look for what
touches your heart, your memories, and
your fears. If one story or one exercise deliv-
ers sudden understanding or amazement
(because you didn't know anyone else
behaved like that), you have found your
entry into your recovery path. I hope this
book supports and sustains you on that path
to freedom. It can be done. I was bulimic

for over twenty-nine years. I've been in recovery for twenty-six years. I've seen and been part of the recovery of many women along the way.

My bulimia story began one summer in New York when I was thirteen years old. I was vacationing at a Catskill Mountains resort with my parents. Guests could order any amount of any food from the dining room menu. I remember men smiling at me and an older woman saying, "Isn't it wonderful how you can eat all those desserts and remain so slim?"

I ordered and ate a sample of all the desserts at every meal. I knew I couldn't get fat because my mother wanted me to win the hotel beauty contest. I didn't want to lose the attention I was getting for my miraculous ability to eat so much, and I knew I had to please my mother by making a good show in the contest.

One night I discovered a secret trick. I could eat heaps of chocolate rugula and tiny creamy pecan pies, and then make myself throw up. Presto! I kept the attention and got rid of the calories. I was elated. I had found the solution to my problem.

The day of the beauty contest arrived, and I felt like a robot going through the motions. When I was on the platform in front of the hotel guests, wearing my white bathing suit, fishnet stockings, and black high heels, I was terrified and felt fat and ugly. Yet against adult women, I won.

I didn't give up my miracle trick after the contest and vacation were over. I continued eating and vomiting all through high school. Except it wasn't a miracle trick anymore; it was something I had to do. It became a shameful secret. I became surreptitious to avoid discovery as I binged and purged.

At first I relied on food at home. I prowled through the refrigerator and ate from leftover containers. I disguised the remains of my secret foraging — leftover stews and pastas were best for this. The uneven and chunky contents didn't show marks of my spoon, the way a slice out of a cake might. Large containers of pudding were also good for the same reason. Individual serving cups of puddings didn't work unless there were many cups. I hoped no one would notice if one or two were missing.

My secret life that was to last almost thirty years had begun. I ate in secret and raided the cupboards and the refrigerator unseen. I took care to leave no trace. I had no money of my own to buy food, so I also had to find subtle ways to binge at the dinner table. I ate slowly and methodically with my family and excused myself in the middle of dinner. I went to the bathroom, drank as much water as I could, jumped up and down to mix it all up inside me, kept the tap running to block my retching sounds, and threw up dinner. Then I rejoined my family at the table and continued to eat.

I struck gold when I started babysitting. The mothers of the children I watched were gracious. After a mother told me what to expect from her child and gave me emergency contact information she would almost always follow with, "If you get hungry, help yourself to a snack." Then she would show me cupboards packed with snack foods and a refrigerator stocked with treats. I believed whole packages of potato chips, crackers, cookies, and ice cream were set out just for the babysitter.

After I put the children to sleep, I'd go to the cupboards and eat everything. Then I'd look for opened packages of food, especially crackers or cereal or cookies. Candy was good too, as long as I could throw it up easily. A limit for me was never opening an unopened package. I remember once seeing a mother who was obviously startled when she noticed how much food was gone. But no one ever said anything. And I was a popular babysitter. I loved the children, played well with them, and was caring and attentive. They always asked for me. It was when the children were asleep that I'd go into my binge/purge dramas.

My attempts to stop my binge/purge episodes through willpower failed within minutes. It never occurred to me to confide in someone or ask for help.

I binged on fruit in an attempt to control my massive eating. I'd take six or more oranges downstairs to the recreation room, turn on the TV, and settle in. First I would peel an orange with a sharp knife. Then, to postpone eating for as long as possible, I would cut the peels into many tiny pieces. I'd cut the white from the orange skin. I tried to get satisfaction from the cutting, but I always moved on to the binge. Looking back, it's curious to me that I never cut myself, as many children and adults suffering from anorexia and bulimia do. That wasn't part of my pattern.

I started college at Northwestern University, where I majored in journalism. At my sorority house, Zeta Tau Alpha, only one bathroom offered privacy. I planned my eating and vomiting so I could use that bathroom when the adjoining room was empty. I binged and threw up before dates in my attempt to appear as a normal eater in public.

I remember long and awkward times in public bathrooms. I risked discovery. If someone came in, they might see my feet turned the wrong way in the stall. In a small public bathroom I risked someone in the adjoining stall hearing me. I couldn't come out until they left. I wonder how much time I spent in bathroom stalls, waiting for people to leave?

My bingeing and purging remained a secret throughout my college years. My attempts to stop were secret, too. I had a sorority sister whose father was a doctor. He gave her a prescription for diet pills, and she often got more than enough to share with her friends. I used amphetamines for two years.

The diet pills did not stop my bingeing and purging. They stunted my hunger pangs, but I never binged or purged because I was hungry. The amphetamines helped me be more methodical in my planning. But the planning itself got out of hand.

The first pill I ever took knocked me out for an hour. When I woke, I felt my blood vibrating in my veins and a new kind of energy that helped me feel unreal and intent on whatever project I had in mind. I gathered my books, my notes, my pads and pens, and began mapping out a complex way to do my work. I became so intent on creating a system that by the time I was ready to actually study, I was too exhausted and confused to get far. I used the pills to stay up all night for several nights in a row studying for finals. No one seemed to think this was abnormal since many of the girls pulled "all-nighters." I wonder how many of us shared similar secrets.

When I realized I was dependent on amphetamines, I stopped taking them and went through withdrawal without knowing the existence of the word, all in secret.

I married when I was twenty. I was living with my parents, and in my mind I was planning an event that was like a play with me in the lead role. I binged and purged three or four times a day and went through the ceremony in a trance. Nothing seemed real — not the groom, not my parents, not me.

My new husband was in the Air Force. We had little money, yet I had to binge and purge. I bought two inexpensive packaged cake mixes at a time, usually lemon cake because I liked it the least and hoped that would slow me down. One night, I baked a cake and served it for dessert. We both had a serving. My husband had another later in the evening.

The next day, after I had devoured the rest of the first cake in secret, I baked the second cake, frosted it, and cut out and ate the equivalent of the three pieces we had eaten the night before so the cake looked the same to my husband. It was the cheapest way to maintain my bulimia. I tried doing this with homemade bread too, but it was too difficult to throw up.

By my early thirties, I was a wife with a teenage daughter, and my life was still unreal. One day, it dawned on me that when my daughter turned eighteen, I'd be forty. These numbers were culturally defined for me. Eighteen meant independence as a girl moved into womanhood. Forty (for women at the time) meant being cast aside as irrelevant. The vision of my life alone with my husband was bleak. I wanted my daughter to become independent, but the thought of my life going on as it was without her to give it meaning was intolerable. I knew I had to prepare myself for the day when she would be on her own, but I didn't know how.

I read classic literature. I volunteered in the community. I binged and purged daily, sometimes up to twelve times a day. My binge/purge episodes kept me busy but provided no relief. I often fell asleep on the couch in front of the TV to stop feeling. When I awoke my despair greeted me. Sometimes I would binge and purge for days, unable to leave the house.

I spent hours on the beach with my German shepherds, Rain and Charlie, because I didn't binge on the beach. I walked and often wrote, but I could not sustain any activity for long. When I realized I could live this way forever, I knew I had to aim for something more. My marriage was lonely, my child was growing up, and I felt I was heading for forty and a drop into oblivion.

I was thirty-two. I decided I would do something to make the day of my fortieth birthday not be just good, but great. My goal was to wake up that morning happy about my life and looking forward to the day. I had no idea how to make that happen. It never occurred to me that I could stop bingeing and throwing up. As I think back, I believe that day was the first time I had a sense of my own future. I could never imagine living more than six months ahead. I believed I would choke to death during a purge. That day it occurred to me that I could take responsibility for my life.

From where I was I reached out to the thing that had been consistently reliable in my life — reading. It had always been my solace, my haven, my escape, and my source of guidance. I enrolled in UCLA, majoring in psychology. I binged and threw up every afternoon. I remember driving home from campus, gripping the steering wheel and saying out loud, "I won't do it." But I always stopped at the market and picked up my chips, ice cream, and Oreo cookies. At home, I ate it all and threw it up.

During my studies at UCLA, I was forced to create boundaries because I needed time and space to learn. I tacked a yellow 8 1/2 × 11-inch sheet of paper above my desk listing all the courses I needed to take in order to graduate with a degree in psychology. It represented two and a half years of work. I looked at that list every day and knew that somehow I had to check off every class if I were going to get to my new life.

Fear or courage, determination or feelings on the edge of despair, drove me on. I had many gaps in my education. I used grammar school, junior high, and high school math textbooks to get me through calculus. A required computer programming course completely baffled me, but a friend helped me through with nightly phone calls and many homework emergency responses.

My life felt grim even as I met the requirements for my schooling, did internships, and studied for licensing exams, while simultaneously experiencing financial loss, raising a teenage daughter, and carrying on a glamorous romance where I lived and breathed the fantasy life of a princess. By the time I was thirty-six and in graduate school, I knew my marriage was over. I binged and purged, drank, and had affairs all throughout the divorce proceedings. This is bulimia in action. I was bingeing, not only on food, but on frantic activity and romance as well.

Between college and graduate school, my husband, daughter, and I went on a family vacation to Cornwall, England. On the trip that was meant to be a bonding experience, I realized I could not pretend there was any life left in my marriage. My husband left England for Los Angeles as we had originally planned. I stayed with my daughter for another week. That's when I met John.

I was still actively bulimic when John made his elegant advances. He fulfilled a bulimic dream I often see in many of my patients as they struggle to open themselves to the first stage of eating disorder recovery. Bulimic fantasies are not compatible with a life in recovery.

John and I had a long distance relationship. I didn't realize he was an alcoholic, even though I noticed his destructive patterns. He didn't know I was bulimic. We saw each other when we were both at our best, and we believed the lies we told each other.

I adored him, and he needed adoration. He treated me royally, which alleviated my terrible feelings of anxiety and worthlessness. We were happy. No, happiness only comes through recovery. We were *ecstatic* and psychologically merged as only two addicts can be.

He took me on extravagant trips around the United Kingdom and through California. We stayed at beautiful hotels, dined on gourmet foods, and built a make-believe future for ourselves. He supported me emotionally through my divorce and the pressures of my graduate studies and professional licensing. I supported him through his medical crisis and a triple bypass heart surgery.

Our relationship fell apart when the fantasies collapsed. Seeing each other intermittently, with all the yearnings and dramas that culminated in sporadic fulfillment, allowed our fantasies to flourish. They faded as we had increasing brushes with the reality of who we were on a full-time basis.

Feast and famine is an underlying theme of eating disorders, and it applies to relationships as well as food. With a healthy commitment to reality, there is no room for relationships based on fantasy and ecstasy. (But, I must admit, I do smile when I remember the ecstasy.)

I binged and purged through all of this. My hair was falling out, and my menses were disrupted. I had a burning discharge the doctors could not diagnose. I look back on this time as the days of peanut butter sandwiches purchased on a flimsy credit card and exquisite lobster dinners in fine restaurants. The contrasts in my life were severe.

Yet, I learned I could get through this (not yet understanding that "this" was my early reaches toward eating disorder recovery). I still didn't know I was bulimic or that eating disorders existed. I knew I had a terrible secret that proved I was a terrible person. But despite seeing myself as a terrible person, I still had managed to shed a bad marriage, get an education, travel, create a better home for my daughter, and keep my promises to her. My daughter stayed in the same high school throughout this time, keeping her routines and friends.

What's remarkable to me is that my compulsive behavior was still a secret. Years later, my husband was shocked when I told him that I was recovering from bulimia during grad school.

The only person who knew was my daughter. Bulimia didn't have a name when I was ill, but my daughter knew when I binged. She knew it was odd for her mother to eat bags of potato chips and sour cream for breakfast in bed. She heard me throwing up in the bathroom sometimes and would knock on the door, asking, "Mommy, Mommy, are you okay?" When I felt dazed and unreal, she felt abandoned.

I did abandon her when I was in those bulimic hazes. I abandoned everyone and everything during those times, including myself. Eating disorder recovery has a lot to do with being present in this life no matter what you have to see, know, and feel. Part of being present now is acknowledging how my oblivion hurt people I love.

Throughout my entire recovery saga runs the ever-present thread of my love for my daughter. Her existence has always been an inspiration to me. One afternoon, long before I was in recovery, I was hiking in the Santa Monica mountains with a young woman who was more wood sprite and mountain goat than human. She led the way through what were familiar trails to her. She was far ahead of me and out of sight when I came to a fearsome place. The trail turned into a tiny stone ledge running between the cliff wall and a drop that was not survivable. I had to put my back against the wall and inch my body along the ledge until I was back again on solid ground. I was sure I couldn't do it. I would have to go back.

Then, I asked myself, "How could I do it?" Beyond the ledge was a large boulder. I said to myself, "What if my daughter was on top of that rock, and tigers were trying to get at her. Would I find a way to get to her?" My answer was a resounding "Yes!" With that image in mind, I got across that ledge.

My plan to have a good life at forty was on schedule. I graduated from my masters program, passed my qualification examinations, and received my Marriage and Family Therapist license. By that time, I was thirty-nine. At forty, my divorce was final, and my daughter was in college.

I liked my life. I had new friends. I found meaning in my work. I could help support my daughter financially and intellectually. I was still bingeing and purging.

Over the years, people have asked me what caused me to stop being bulimic. I have different answers as I continue on my journey. Certainly my awareness that my daughter's eighteenth birthday would coincide with my fortieth woke me up. I began understanding that my child's life had a trajectory. I couldn't imagine a long life for myself, but I became invested in my daughter's growth and development. I expected her to live, develop, and have a future. And when I imagined her living an independent life, I discovered I wanted a long future for myself, too. I didn't want to leave her. So my first step into recovery, (although I didn't know it) was to believe I had a future. Then my recovery work began. Another awakening thought occurred to me one day. While checking my reflection in the bathroom mirror for any telltale spatter from my purge, I thought, "What if I used all the energy I put into my eating disorder for something else? What might I accomplish in life?" It occurred to me, for the first time, that maybe I had a choice about bingeing and purging.

I believe that was the conscious start of my recovery. The people who were most influential in holding me, teaching me, loving me, guiding me, and providing me with therapy and inspiration were already in my life. I had made choices, unconsciously, that put who and what I needed near me, wonderful, trustworthy, and capable people to support me.

My former clinical supervisor, Lars Lofgren, included me in his family. Lars and his wife, Ingeborg, became my loving, grounded, and elegant home base for Sunday dinners, talks by the fire, and honest sharing. A recovering alcoholic psychiatrist I'll call Michael, became a teacher and mentor as I worked my way through 12-step groups finding my path.

Hedda Bolgar accepted me in her practice and, through her love, skill, and the powers of psychoanalysis, helped me clear psychological rubble blocking my way to recovery.

The requirements of my profession gave me opportunities to practice what I was learning in classes, seminars, group trainings, and readings. I shared work with colleagues at the UCLA Neuropsychiatric Institute as we studied guided imagery and helped one another learn to help others and ourselves. I stopped being locked into a false presentation of who I was and began living a life that gave me the opportunity to build a real person — me.

Because I was ill, I was a flawed mother. But like so many mothers I see in my practice today, I was determined to make a good life possible for my daughter. Moving toward recovery and well-being for myself created a better life for both of us. I earned enough money to provide a lovely home near her school and friends, which had seemed impossible only a year earlier. I developed myself, my career, and my new friendships in order to be a better person for me and a more positive influence in her life. I'm happy to say she lives her satisfying and fulfilling life today. Love is a powerful motivating force.

I didn't intend to specialize in working with women who had eating disorders, but I kept following my heart and my authentic values as I learned to recognize them. As I healed and developed, I studied and spoke about what interested me and what I cared about. I discovered that there was more to me than being a woman with an eating disorder, as I had believed when in the depth of my illness. I discovered that women in their thirties, forties, fifties, and sixties were revealing their eating disorders as more of us spoke openly about our lives. I came to believe I had value to offer.

Today my goal is to help others who are suffering from eating disorders to achieve health and freedom. I believe that healing, developing the person you authentically are, and honoring your heart frees you from terrible fears that make eating disorders necessary. Further, I'm confident that your recovery exerts a healing influence on others.

Living with an eating disorder is a miserable way to live. Women often live with their eating disorders for many years before seeking help. Stopping the behavior is good, but it's not enough. I've heard women say, (and I've said it too), "I want my life to have meaning." We don't want those years consumed by an eating disorder to be lost years. We want to go beyond recovery into a life that is worth living. With recovery comes a unique awareness and knowledge we never would have had without struggling with an eating disorder. When we find value in that knowledge, we are truly in recovery and in a life that is satisfying and free.

I wrote this book, word after word, in a linear fashion because that's how books get written. But you are not linear. Each chapter describes a particular issue that requires skills, growth, understanding, and courage to negotiate. As a nonlinear human being, you will most likely be confronted with many of your personal issues at the same time. Please do not be dismayed. Every chapter is designed to help you develop the awareness, self-compassion, and tools to keep you moving on your recovery path. Each bit of growth and healing you experience will help you in all phases of your life. The chapters are designed to help you build, layer upon layer, the means to nourish your own health and become less afraid, less bewildered, and more present and more capable.

Please remember, helping yourself does not mean going it alone. Helping yourself means committing to your life and supporting your own recovery. This includes learning how to recognize opportunity and reach out to people who are in a position to offer you genuine help on your journey to healing. Part of recovery is learning how to make wise choices about trustworthy and honorable people. They will come.

A happy — an amazing — surprise awaits you in recovery. Your goal may be to lose weight or lose your obsession. You may yearn to escape your fears and feel safe. You can't imagine more than that. In recovery, you discover that you can be more alive than you ever dreamed. You discover that trustworthy people honor you, welcome your gifts, support your endeavors, and even offer you love. You learn that you are valuable and can find joy in sharing the gift of yourself. What's more, you learn to recognize love and not accept false substitutes. You become present in the world as a real woman.

CHAPTER 2
BEGINNING TO FREE YOURSELF

"In the truest sense, freedom cannot be bestowed; it must be achieved."
— Franklin D. Roosevelt

Before you picked up this book, you probably looked for ways to recover many times. Maybe some of your methods were questionable: You tried diets to lose weight; you chewed sugarless gum until your jaw ached; you may have tried drugs to squelch your appetite or control your feelings. Maybe you surrendered to your eating disorder and isolated yourself with TV and binge food as your main companions. In public, you may have hidden your too-thin or too-fat or just plain unacceptable body in layers of clothing, smiled a smile you didn't mean, and kept yourself so busy you didn't have time to know what you were feeling. You may have distracted eyes from your rotund or skeletal body by wearing expensive or flamboyant jewelry.

When these tricks succeeded, you felt safe as eyes bounced off you and moved on, or if you beguiled those eyes with accessories. At the same time, you were not happy being treated as if you were invisible or when someone focused on your embellishments. You created a barrier between yourself and other people so that having a genuine relationship was an unlikely possibility. This "success" caused you much loneliness.

Now, book in hand, you are ready to explore a path that might be new for you — and it might work. You want to be free. You share this desire with all men and women who are dependent on an eating disorder.

Most of the people I work with are women, so I use the feminine pronoun in this book. I'm reporting the details of the successful treatment of women in my practice over the years, plus my own recovery story. When you, man or woman, focus on the personal details of your life and understand how you act out your eating disorder, you have the potential to move toward your recovery and heal. Are you ready to begin?

Research about eating disorders continues at all levels of psychology and medicine, dispelling myths and gathering new information. (See Appendix C for findings and summaries.) Yet many of the ideas and information about eating disorders, even when based on credible ongoing research, are still controversial.

Eating disorders have the highest mortality rate of any mental disorder. Bingeing and purging plays havoc with teeth and gums and can harm the esophagus, and over extended periods of time it disrupts electrolytes in the body, which can result in a heart attack. Anorexia leads to heart problems, infertility, and osteoporosis.

Some people might suffer from bulimia and anorexia without having complicating medical problems. Some live long lives. I've known anorexic women in their eighties, bent over with osteoporosis and suffering from mild to moderate dementia. I remember Bella, frail and thin at eighty-five. Her osteoporosis created a "hump" in her back that pushed her upper torso forward. I watched her buttoning her cardigan sweater. Because of the angle of her body, the buttons and button holes didn't connect. In a harsh staccato voice she said, "I'm so fat. Damn it. I'm not eating today." My breath stopped. My chest ached as I stood witness to the ravaged leavings of a lifetime of anorexia. Bella no longer had a choice, but you do.

This book lays out essential guidelines for creating and supporting your ongoing recovery. As you move through the chapters, you will learn how to choose or create the exercises and activities that are right for you. You and I are collaborators in this process. Each chapter lays the groundwork for exploring your emotions and experiences at tolerable levels of intensity. As you develop the emotional capacity to be present, you will grow beyond your suffering. You *can* be known and understood.

The following list of experiences may not seem, on the surface, to relate to eating disorders. Most of them are not specifically about food or eating. But they can reveal how you use your eating disorder to live behind a façade. In responding to the list below, please use the words *never, rarely, sometimes, often,* or *always.*

1. I hide from people.
2. I've thought about suicide.
3. I find it difficult or impossible to make long range commitments.
4. I have emotional meltdowns where I am terrified and feel lost.
5. I have a disappointing — and somewhat shameful and secret — sex life.

6. I feel a low, continuous anger and resentment towards people in my life.
7. My short-term memory doesn't function well.
8. I say to myself "This is the last time I will _____" about certain behaviors but invariably repeat them.
9. I describe my suffering to someone and ask for help, yet reject suggestions offered.
10. I perform relentless exercise routines to ward off caloric consequences.
11. I eat mindlessly when I'm not hungry.
12. I tell lies at the grocery store checkout stand when buying my binge foods.
13. I weigh myself every day or several times a day.

Please breathe and know that you have just completed a powerful task. You might feel anxious or relieved. You may think you are overwhelmed, but you are not. You may be surprised or dismayed to discover how many of these descriptions apply to you and how much time they take up in your life. You may begin to criticize yourself or feel terribly deficient. But please put aside self-punishing thoughts. You are simply beginning to take a first look at the reality of your life, especially those aspects dominated by your eating disorder.

If you have had any of the experiences in this list, you have to live this way. Let's acknowledge that strength right now. Fortitude, creativity, determination, and strategic thinking are required to maintain an eating disorder and all of its demands. If you have the strength and ability to sustain an eating disorder, then you have the strength and ability to move beyond it. Together, we have a chance to find a way out of your torment and into a much healthier and happier way of living.

Your honest response to the questions in the list will alert you to areas in your life that need support, love, care, healing, and encouragement. When you finish going over the list, create a recovery journal with a separate page for each item that applies to you. These pages will provide topics of your choosing for journal entries, free writing, and explorations. Instead of eating or starving, or relying on food or excessive exercise to give you safety and emotional numbing, your journaling on these topics will help you heal your way through your troubling experiences, ultimately making your eating disorder unnecessary.

Sometimes your feelings will come up so fast you seem to have no choice except to act out your eating disorder. Often, you don't know you are feeling anything. You follow an irresistible urge to eat, or you discover yourself eating without being aware of when you started. You might, for example, find yourself eating your child's unfinished lunch in the kitchen before you wash the plate. You might notice that the one cookie you ate from the dish on the coffee table led to your eating all the cookies. You may or may not have noticed the surprise on the faces of people who saw you.

When you are in the grip of your urges, you have emotional tunnel vision. It's difficult or impossible for you to imagine options. You are not aware of the consequences of your behavior to your health, your use of time, and your relationships.

At the close of each chapter, you'll find exercises based on the healing benefits of mindful breathing, affirmations, and writing that will help you expand your mind and develop your ability to move beyond the dictates of your eating disorder. They will become more involved as you progress on your recovery path. To start, here's a description of what to expect and what to try first.

BREATHING

Breathing and noticing the details of your breath flow will help you to unite your sense of yourself and stay present in the moment. Stopping your activity and attending to your breath throughout the day, regardless of urges, cravings, or powerful emotions will gently and subtly build a pathway for you to be present without needing your eating disorder.

Give yourself a minimum of five minutes to quietly watch your breath. Breathe normally. Watch where your breath starts. Notice when you feel your breath in your lungs or nose or throat. Notice when you lose track of it. You cannot make a mistake here, you simply attend to your breath *as it is.* Do this at least three times in a twenty-four-hour period.

Because you are bright and because you want results quickly, you might try to make more of this exercise than what I describe here. For example, you might think you are supposed to be thinking some particular thing or you are supposed to get some kind of revelation or inspiration by attending to your breath. Not so. Attending to your breath is a building block for your recovery. You may extend the time if you wish. But, please, keep it simple.

AFFIRMATIONS

It takes a month or two of practicing a new behavior to change a habit or mindset. Repeating self-affirming statements along the way helps you accept your developing strengths and self-knowledge.

Choose three affirmations you believe would make your life better. For example: "I enjoy excellent help," "I am lovable," and "I succeed where I put my efforts." Read each aloud twenty times each morning, noon, and night. Change your position as you read: stand in one place with correct posture; walk around a room or outdoors; stand before a mirror.

At the end of one month, add new affirmations to your list. You may substitute them for the affirmations you did the preceding month, or you may tack them on to your first month's list. See Appendix A for more affirmations and advice for creating your own.

JOURNALING

Almost every self-help book suggests some form of writing. You've probably had some experience in journaling or keeping a diary. You may even keep a journal now.

When you pour your thoughts and feelings onto the page, you are able to see them more clearly. The page holds your written thoughts and feelings, not you. You become free to read, observe, think, and feel something other than what you wrote.

This is particularly helpful when you are in the thick of an emotional storm or when you have a difficult decision to make. You can write your dilemma onto the page and then ask for what you want and need. You might be surprised to discover that after you write out your problem and ask for help, your own psyche, or the voice of your heart and soul, comes through with relevant answers. In your recovery work, you'll harness the power of journaling to help you clear entrenched false beliefs and automatic responses and behaviors so you are free to discover new and more self-caring options.

At this early stage in your journaling, you can write anything. You'll fine tune your writing later on. Right now your first step is to befriend pen and paper. Write at least three pages every day about anything you want. Complain. Fantasize. Write down your plans for the next hour or week or lifetime. Describe people in your life or the room you are in. Write at home, in the park, in your car, in a waiting room, at a café, on a bus bench. Just write three pages.

Think of your journal as a camera, writing descriptions of what you see, or a tape recorder, writing about what you hear.

In Appendix D, "Recovery Journal Prompts," you will find additional topics to journal on. Build gradually toward journaling on these topics. Right now, simply free write and see what happens. Give yourself the gift of letting your heart and mind release what you've been holding, and give yourself room to breathe and be just as you are.

The chapters that follow will give you examples of the experiences of women living with and recovering from eating disorders, as well as exercises, stories, and meditations that will provide you with a lifeline to grow out of current painful and destructive ways.

Please pace yourself. Part of living with an eating disorder is wanting and grasping for immediate gratification. (One sugary doughnut or a dozen can knock out feelings. It's only natural that you would hope for a fast route to recovery.) Part of living with an eating disorder means you believe you are not doing enough, are not good

44

enough or fast enough. This book is full of things to do. But you don't have to do them all, and you certainly don't have to do them all at once. Let your recovery unfold at a pace you can sustain. Recovery is not a sprint. You are going for the long distance of your life.

Please, proceed gently with yourself. Recovery comes in layers and stages, with pauses in between to settle. Think of the layering Rembrandt used in his master-pieces. (Yes, you are a masterpiece too.) He painted meticulously with oils. Then he waited until a layer was completely dry and absorbed by the canvas before he added the next layer. He gave himself and the painting time to breathe and acclimate to new stages. So must you.

Through gradual and regular practice, you will develop a strength and stability that you can't imagine now. As you proceed, you will discover how to be present and capable of coping with your challenges. Your fears will diminish as you progress on your recovery path.

DAILY EXERCISES

Remember to pace yourself. The exercises and activities listed below and in Appendix B,

"Additional Exercises and Activities," will gradually expand as you gain strength. They will help steady and support you as we take a closer look at your life in the next chapter.

1. Follow your breath for five minutes at least three times a day.
2. Read or recite three affirmations twenty times each, at least three times a day. See Appendix A, "Affirmations."
3. Write a minimum of three pages in your journal each day.

CHAPTER 3
EARLY WARNING SIGNS

"Every patient carries her or his own
doctor inside."
— Albert Schweitzer

This chapter goes more deeply into how you live and what needs your attention. What follows are possible early warning signs of an eating disorder or behaviors that, when repeated, can indicate an ongoing eating disorder. Be gentle with yourself as you examine the things you consider normal and routine, but which may indicate a serious problem.

You benefit from reviewing the way you live. How you behave with and around food, how you eat and do not eat, and the habits and idiosyncrasies you've developed around eating relate to the full scope of your life. For example, if you binge on food, you may also binge on people, or clothes, or drama. If you purge, you may feel clean and powerful when you throw away objects, leave gatherings, or end relationships. If you starve yourself, you may also restrict emotional nourishment and deprive yourself of money, education, and the opportunity for healthy relationships. If you feel proud when you refuse food, you may feel proud when you refuse assistance or opportunities to better your life.

Once you have an accurate picture of your eating disorder, you have a window into the patterns of your emotions and psychology. You also — and this is important — can use your eating disorder behaviors as a metaphor to understand how you behave in other situations. This is the beginning of making your eating disorder a valuable life teacher.

Your first and ongoing challenge is to not judge yourself. Merciless self-condemnation is a symptom of an eating disorder. You may have people in place who do that for you — that's another sign. If you can't resist criticizing yourself, give yourself a time limit to do so, and then do your breathing exercises. A brief mindful breathing practice after a bout of self criticism can help you realign yourself with self-kindness.

Defining unusual eating behaviors is a challenge, because what's considered normal keeps changing in our culture. Unfortunately, this difficulty makes it easier for early warning signs of an eating disorder to be missed, denied, or rationalized. Today, eating disorders not otherwise specified (EDNOS) cover more of the population than identified eating disorders. Disordered eating, emotional eating, binge eating, or occasional purging may qualify as EDNOS. For recovery purposes, look at any form of eating that seems disordered and that troubles you, causes you problems, or is essential for you to cope with unbearable feelings.

In the not-so-distant past, taking time to sit at a dining table and eat three meals a day at a slow and gentle pace was normal. Now, grabbing a smoothie for breakfast while you dash for the car, rushing through a twenty-minute lunch "hour," or ordering Chinese food and then eating it from the container with a group of friends are not extraordinary or bizarre activities today. Living on fast food may not be part of a healthy lifestyle, but it doesn't necessarily signal an eating disorder.

Eating a peanut butter sandwich for breakfast and having pancakes or scrambled eggs for dinner is not unusual in a fast-paced urban life, nor does it signal an eating disorder. Eating leftovers for breakfast doesn't indicate an eating disorder, either. Such behavior may mean the food is convenient when you are in a hurry or that you liked it and are eager to have more before it spoils. It could also mean that you are being economical by not wasting food.

Similarly, it's possible to have a seemingly healthy diet and suffer from an eating disorder. For example, in the past decade, the term "slow food" has entered the mainstream American vocabulary. Growing your own food or shopping at farmers' markets for items you will cook slowly at home can enrich family life, enhance health, and help the environment. Eating slow food, however, doesn't mean you don't have an eating disorder.

Unusual eating behaviors that indicate a problem might include: hiding food so you won't be tempted to eat it, but then becoming frantic when you can't find it in your usual hiding places or can't remember if you ate it already. Frantic, you suck on raw sugar cubes, drink maple syrup from the bottle, or find a bottle of chocolate sauce and drink it straight. None of this soothes as well as your binge food, but you feel a little more calm. You also feel terribly ashamed. And now the kitchen is a mess, and you're anxious because you've got to cover your tracks.

Another indication is when you finish food that is partially eaten, like a container of ice cream. Then you replace the carton with another that is the same size, brand, and flavor, eating from it until the amount of ice cream matches the original before you took any.

You may pour hot sauce or hot spices on your food, not because you like the spices, but so the food will burn your mouth and throat and stomach. You hope that the pain involved with every bite will slow down your ability to binge or stop you completely. If any of these examples sound familiar to you, you have an eating disorder.

Eating disorder indications take many forms. You cut food into many tiny pieces. You feel busy, thoroughly occupied, and safe for the moment while you are cutting because you are close to food but not eating. When you are eating with others you spit food into your napkin and hide it under your plate. You are angry or anxious if someone comments on what you are eating.

Appetite control drugs won't stop this kind of behavior, because you are not reacting to food on the basis of physical hunger. When you see what may be your own episodes articulated, you are more likely to sense the anguish and almost blind fear and desperation behind the behavior. Awareness of proper nutrition and portion size for a healthy body is irrelevant to your needs on these occasions. Strict dieting only pulls back these urges like a sling shot. As your fears and tensions build, you snap back into an even more voracious binge episode with or without purging.

If you are anorexic, you may starve for long periods of time and then break through with a binge that would amaze even a bulimic woman. The purging afterwards can bring up blood as well as food. You might pass out.

Internally, you may feel like you're warding off an incoming dark, rolling thundercloud that could destroy you unless you reach for your eating disorder behavior. Recovery is about developing ways to cope with such feelings without resorting to self-destructive behavior.

I often tell a new client that I'm not going to take her eating disorder away. I can't. I don't know how, and even if I did know how, I wouldn't. It's serving a purpose. To strip your eating disorder away would leave you exposed and vulnerable to your unbearable fears with no protection. It would be like taking off your armor in the middle of a battle. Yes, the armor is heavy. You are hot and sticky in there. You can't move quickly. You could drown in a stream. You can't touch another person or feel another's touch. But the armor does protect you from arrows and spears that are coming at you from all directions. You take off armor when you can take care of yourself. Then the benefits of your defense outweigh the discomforts and risks. You seek recovery work when you realize the eating disorder you rely on to soothe you is causing more suffering than you can accept. Or you seek recovery when your eating disorder fails and you can no longer use it for emotional relief.

As you recognize symptoms and situations that relate to your eating disorder and understand that they are not fundamental to your nature, you develop more distance and more curiosity about them. This helps you be more gentle and patient with yourself. When your self-criticism diminishes, you are free to take new recovery steps.

You may discover you have unusual attitudes about food. Some foods may seem to have the power to call out with emotional messages, memories, promises, threats, joys, or dangers. Perhaps pasta, pancakes, Asian noodles, popcorn, or ice cream seem to promise you a safe haven. You can eat these foods and be comforted. Perhaps chocolate kisses or chocolate-covered cherries or thick grilled cheese sandwiches, or bananas with peanut butter, or whole jars of olives, or bread heavily laden with melted butter were family favorites and indulgences when you were a child. Perhaps your family had lovely private times together while eating these foods. Thus, they call to you when you are craving safety or intimacy — or maybe they frighten you for the same reason. The glitch in your system that creates the eating disorder is that you go for the symbol rather than the real thing. If you don't know a realistic way to bring safety and ease into your life, you may eat or starve to reach your personal safe haven.

You may have a loved one in your life who also has difficulties with food. He or she may encourage you to eat more than is healthy and satisfying for you or less than is adequate to sustain a healthy weight.

Nora, fifty-five, has suffered from compulsive overeating since she was a teenager. When she was a teen, her mother criticized her for being fat during the day but secretly gave her deep-fried peanut butter sandwiches and chocolate shakes at night when everyone had gone to bed. Nora liked the experience of kindness and intimacy with her mother during those times. Now, without realizing it, she tries to reclaim that sense of being loved through food.

Sylvia, twenty-three, said she had no control or influence over her finances and lived with her aunt, who locked the refrigerators and cupboards and carefully monitored Sylvia's eating allowance — small portions of inexpensive food — while the aunt ate normally. Sylvia, very thin, suffered from a kind of anorexia. She was caught in a system that perpetuated the eating disorder. Away from that environment, when a friend offered her food, she was afraid to eat, afraid of being punished for disobeying the rules she believed she must live by.

One afternoon, while I was grocery shopping, I saw a young woman I knew shopping with her mother. Martha was EDNOS with strong anorexic symptoms. She didn't see me, and her mother didn't know me. The pair was hovering over a fruit display. I saw Martha caress apples, bananas, and mangos and look questioningly at her mother. Her mother frowned and shook her head. Martha, carrying an empty shopping basket, like a beggar woman hoping for crumbs, walked alongside her mother as she filled her cart with food that was destined for a locked refrigerator.

Martha, though intelligent and creative, didn't have a sturdy enough psyche to create a life of her own where she could earn her own money to buy and eat her own food. She was well educated, but she had been sexually molested regularly and was physically abused as a young child. Her mother, perhaps unaware of her jealousy and rage, treated her like an unwanted captive. Her distant father considered her a sexual toy. The young woman's heart, spirit, and ability to be her true self were locked away in a psychological prison long ago. She didn't have access to a way out yet.

Martha haunts me. I wonder how many women are like her. What doorway or window, or glimmer of light, could reach through her interior prison so she could begin to move toward recovery as I hope you are doing? Maybe she is reading this book.

Cooking masses of food for family and friends or as a caterer, yet not eating anything yourself, is another warning sign. Carolyn, forty-seven and a working professional, watched friends eat food she longed to eat herself. She used all the control she could muster to deny herself the nourishment she craved and her body needed. She felt proud of her success in not eating.

Carolyn needed to maintain a sense of superiority over other people. She believed she could live without what she considered to be mundane needs for physical nourishment. She felt others were stuck in heavy body prisons while she was moving beyond the need of her slight frame. She was striving to be perfect, a pure spirit with no need for the gross consumption of food. She used the words, "It will make me fat" frequently, but her real fear was that food would make her solid and present and part of the human community. If that happened, she wouldn't be able to find safety through her pursuit of being light, untouchable, and perfect. This issue of striving for self-defined perfection will come up again in future chapters.

Cleo, forty-two, looked at foods with a sauce as dangerous because they might taste good. She feared that if she took one mouthful of a food that tasted good to her, she would have no control, eat too much, and get fat before she left the table. Cleo behaved as if her imagined fear was a real threat. She believed if she reached for something she desired, she would lose all control. Cleo not only denied herself food but also intimate relationships, career opportunities, and even simple items to decorate her home. Her walls were bare.

I remember speaking to an emaciated woman lying in a UCLA hospital bed, dying of starvation. She was asking for help and said she wanted to live, but she wouldn't let the doctors give her a feeding tube because, she said, "They all want to make me fat." The tragedy is that the extreme of this distorted thinking ends in death.

Another unusual attitude about food results in weight gain rather than thinness. Food can seem dangerous if you are hungry. You then become more afraid of feeling hungry than of the food. If you graze continually throughout the day, especially on high fat/high sugar snacks, you can assure yourself of never being hungry. Then you have a sense of being in control even though you are frustrated and miserable as your weight continually climbs.

Fear permeates these examples, and fear needs to be addressed more than the food itself.

Further complicating matters, a starved body also means a starved brain. A starved brain creates a mind that cannot think clearly and is subject to wild distortions. It's important to remember that a heavy person can have a starved brain as well as a thin person.

If you have an eating disorder, you ignore the genuine needs of your body. Yet, your body is real, and the human body needs adequate nourishment to function. Adequate nourishment becomes part of recovery, yet it has to be approached with caution since you will experience any change in your eating habits as tampering with what keeps you safe in this world.

You control your moods and experience by eating the foods you have learned "work" for you. For example, you can eat several handfuls of nuts or some fruit and cheese before you go out to dinner with other people. By eating this heavy food, you protect yourself against feeling hunger in public. You protect yourself from feeling out of control, vulnerable, or natural with your companions. You can choose what you will eat and feel comfortable.

This may or may not be a problem. Only you know if this is troublesome for you. If you need to binge and purge before a social dinner, you have a problem.

If you know you will be eating with people who delay the meal beyond your comfort zone, it makes sense to eat beforehand so you aren't too famished. But if you are

59

unwilling to allow others to see you when you feel something authentic, including hunger, then you are eating in advance for protection.

Emotional eating presents a dilemma if you eat to relieve tension even though your stomach is quite full. You might eat on a full stomach and cause yourself pain so you can't participate in activities. Or maybe you eat on a full stomach and throw up. Hours on a treadmill might take care of those calories, but running while your stomach is overloaded can create digestive problems.

Eating until you are so full you pass out is an indication of a possible eating disorder. If you do this to relieve stress, you make yourself non-functional. You have to cancel appointments, miss opportunities, and are unavailable to friends and family. Trying to get through emotional strain by chewing packs of sugar-free gum is an attempt to get binge eating relief without eating. The excessive chewing can cause gas, painful gastric distress, and embarrassing diarrhea. If and when these complications occur, they only add to your sense of shame and worthlessness.

The ultimate goal of a woman in the grip of severe anorexia is to disappear, to lose her body completely, to not only be as light as air, but to actually be air. This dangerous goal gets mixed up with spirituality. The anorexic woman wants to be "pure spirit," gossamer in the wind. If she could reach this impossible ultimate fantasy, she would be invisible to the human eye and sensed only as a vibrating energy that others could feel but not see. If this is you, please know that in your attempt to reach such a goal, you can starve yourself into emaciation, organ destruction, and loss of brain function. If you continue striving for this "ultimate" goal, you will die.

A different anorexia scenario involves separating your sense of self from your body. If you achieve this psychological split, you create an experience where you send your body into the world while your real self remains unknown. You become a puppeteer moving the strings of your body, manipulating it to be the shape required and to function as needed. This, I believe, is part of the dynamic for anorexic women who need or want to be thin for public display.

Yet another addition to these scenarios is believing you feel anxious and bad about yourself because your body is fat, ugly, and disgusting, irrespective of your actual appearance. You use the words "fat" and "ugly" interchangeably. You believe you would feel better, even wonderful, if you were beautiful. Again, you try to use your physicality to tend to your emotional needs, usually at the price of a healthy body.

I've worked with celebrities whose beauty is acclaimed by thousands, even millions, yet who still say they feel fat and ugly. Such a woman knows that her appearance wields power in her world. She may use her beauty as a negotiating tool or as a way of influencing or manipulating. She may consider people influenced by her appearance to be fools because they don't see the frightened, helpless, ugly, fat, and unlovable person she believes herself to be. She's in a complex and painful state. She's won because her true self is invisible. She's lost because she's alone with her ever-present, self-punishing inner voice.

A woman who suffers from binge eating or bulimia can also believe she has the power to make herself invisible. The need to isolate is part of all eating disorders to some degree.

When Kimberly, twenty-nine and suffering from bulimia, needed her binge foods, she put on her "invisible clothes," usually innocuous sweatpants and sweatshirt and a blank look on her face, and got herself to a grocery store or take-out restaurant. She didn't look anyone in the eye. She avoided personal connection and felt that she was a shadow figure who couldn't be seen. If she saw someone she knew, she made it clear with body language that she didn't see or recognize them. If the person didn't respond to her, it reinforced her belief that she was invisible.

When Kimberly got home she rushed through putting away the perishables, leaving out the boxes and bags of salty, crunchy, and sweet. She gathered up her binge foods and felt relief that she could give up the strain of being invisible and get on with eating, secure in her sense of being alone in her private and unseen world.

Janet, forty-five, achieved her invisibility by using what she considered sleight of hand. In public she ate small and seemingly inconsequential tidbits she was certain no one would notice. While other people filled their plates or nibbled on appetizers, Janet was stealing. She took candy decorations from food trays when she believed no one was looking and quickly popped them in her mouth. She also filled her pockets and her purse with sweets to eat on the way home.

A very large woman knows about yet

another kind of invisibility. She can be still and disappear into the background. I remember attending a crowded Overeaters Anonymous meeting of about 200 people. Men and women of all ages and sizes sat in rows of chairs. Those who couldn't find a seat sat on the floor or stood along the walls.

I sat in a chair near a thick pole for at least twenty minutes before I realized a woman was standing in front of that pole. She seemed to gradually appear. She must have weighed close to 350 pounds. She wore a loose-fitting garment in shades of brown and stood immobile and expressionless.

After I noticed her, I looked around the room again. I saw four more women, large, immobile, expressionless, in bland neutral colors, whom I hadn't seen before. I wondered how many women I had never noticed; how much I played into the invisibility mechanism by accepting their unspoken communication: "Don't see me."

Recovery involves becoming visible, ending isolation, and coming out from behind a barrier that protects you from exposure, criticism, reality, friends, opportunities, love, and hope — a barrier that blocks you from life itself.

Another warning sign of an eating disorder is striving for perfection. I'm not referring to the perfection a scientist seeks in conducting valid and reliable research. I mean the kind of perfection where you need to have the perfect body and are miserable and self-critical if you fall short; where you need to create the perfect environment or be the perfect person at your job, at school, or in your family and feel an inner disaster if you fall short. If you can't focus on a relationship, a conversation, or an activity because your mind is busy figuring out ways to make something in your life perfect, you are experiencing warning signs of an eating disorder.

Why? What is it about perfection? Why is a bulimic woman merciless in her self-criticism? Why is an anorexic woman so driven to be perfect she is willing to face death? Why do women who binge or eat compulsively feel so removed from acceptability and standards of perfection that they numb themselves to emotional pain and function tangentially in the world as they attempt to be unseen?

Perfection is the ultimate safety. When anything is perfect, it is beyond criticism, beyond judgment. But perfection, for us mortals, is impossible to achieve. In Greek mythology, whenever a mortal attempted to achieve the status of a god or even one quality of a god, the mortal was cursed and went mad or died. The lesson: Humans aren't designed to be perfect. Perfection is for the gods.

Recovery begins as you venture toward being kind and honest with your genuine, mortal self. You may be ready to be in a room with other people who are working toward recovery, or you may need to be more private as you begin your healing efforts. Respect your feelings. You can begin to move on your healing path through the suggestions in this book — doing affirmations, breathing exercises, and writing in a Recovery Journal. See more specific exercises and activities related to this chapter in Appendix B.

My goal is to help you build a solid recovery, layer by layer. Beginning this journey requires courage. You are changing direction. You are opening your mind and heart to what you don't know yet. Courage and trust are a vital part of recovery work because you don't yet have a backlog of successes on which to build your confidence. You're going on faith, hope, and courage now. Honor and nurture those qualities. Go gently into the unknown, building as you go.

I've described many forms an eating

disorder can take, but not all. Yet enough is here to help you see how much of your life and your behaviors are determined by eating or not eating. Please congratulate yourself for staying with this reconnaissance and getting a more thorough sense of where you are and what needs to be addressed to get well. This is a tender time.

DAILY EXERCISES

1. Follow your breath for five minutes at least three times a day.
2. Read or recite your three affirmations twenty times each at least three times a day. See Appendix A, "Affirmations."
3. Write about one or more of the warning signs discussed in this chapter or a personal experience where you recognized eating disorder signals.

CHAPTER 4
HOW DO I BEGIN RECOVERY?

"What will open the door is daily
awareness and attention."
— Krishnamurti

You've already begun your recovery by picking up this book. Perhaps you are reading it thoroughly, going through each chapter, doing the suggested exercises, and have now come to chapter four. You are on your way.

Perhaps you are standing in a bookstore thumbing through pages and stopped at this chapter. You are reading what I'm writing right now. I'm thinking about you and imagining you as you stand in the aisle or sit in one of those hard-to-find cushy chairs against the wall. You want recovery. Maybe you are holding this book carefully so no one can see the title. Recovery seems secretive, magical, out of reach, mysterious, and impossible because you've tried many times and failed.

Wherever you are right now, if you can see these words, you are looking for your beginning place. The good news is that you can begin any time, at any stage in your life, and in any situation or circumstance.

I wish I could help you take a breath or jump up and down with you and shout to the world, "I don't care what anyone thinks. I don't care about your judgments. I have an eating disorder. I will do whatever it takes to recover, and I don't care who knows it!"

That kind of verve will come after some progress in your recovery work. You begin at your beginning. I've often wondered where my beginning place was. I've had many that qualify.

When I was still immersed in my secret bulimic way of living I attended a small dinner party at the home of my close friends, Lars and Ingeborg. As I mentioned earlier, that night I met a recovering alcoholic psychiatrist I'll call Michael, who invited me to lead a guided imagery session, my specialty at the time, with his alcoholic patients.

I said I didn't know if I could because I didn't know anything about alcoholics. I didn't know yet that I had had a long relationship with an alcoholic, or that some aspects of my bulimia had a great deal in common with alcoholism.

Michael took me to my first AA meeting. I listened to one young man open his heart and with raw honesty describe his daily physical and emotional life as an alcoholic. I was stunned as, for the first time, I heard my secret life described in detail. My life was exactly like his except my issue was food, not alcohol.

I said nothing to Michael but ventured into Overeaters Anonymous where, another first for me, I met a woman who was bulimic and told me so. This was another staggering experience. I whispered to her that I was, too. She nodded and swept away, but I didn't feel rejected. I felt amazed that I wasn't the only one and that I could speak of it.

I started psychotherapy. My clinical supervisor, Hedda Bolgar, agreed to accept me as her patient. I moved through massive fear to tell her I was bulimic. I was prepared for her to reject me and also tell me I could no longer be a psychotherapist. But her face was kind as she welcomed me and we began our journey.

At a private dinner I confessed to Michael that I was bulimic and starting recovery. I expected to see revulsion on his face.

Instead, he smiled and wept. He put his hands together in a silent prayer and said, "It's God's grace." He said my new beginning reinforced his own recovery. I cried too.

A few days later I spent a long Sunday with Lars and Ingeborg, who had given the dinner party where I met Michael. Finally, at a table in a darkened restaurant, I mustered enough courage to tell them I was bulimic. Ingeborg looked blank and asked me what that was. I breathed deeply and described my secret life. She took my hands in hers and said, "We love you, Joanna. How sad for you." Lars smiled a little smile and said, "Joanna, you are the most interesting person."

Was this my starting point? I certainly thought so. But I had already chosen these people to be in my life. I created the opportunity for those events to happen long before I knew how they would turn out. In the film *Field of Dreams,* a voice says, "Build it, and they will come." Buddhism says, "Create the right conditions." Psychotherapy teaches, "Create a sturdy holding environment because we never know what will emerge during the course of treatment."

Bringing this book into your life is part of creating the right conditions for your recovery. What else do you need?

Rather than decide intellectually at this point, take a look at where you are now and what you want. This creates the "right conditions" for your imagination, emotions, and thoughts to come together to make choices that serve you well in the here and now. Then, you can bring your energy to whatever task you decide to undertake.

This sounds vague because I'm not telling you what to choose. You choose. You are the only person who has accurate knowledge about your daily experiences and access to your own authentic visions for yourself. You can check in with your emotions, energy, and courage to start at your true beginning place. You are reading this book because somewhere inside of you, despite the grip of your eating disorder, you want to be free. Your challenge now is to honor and nurture that hopeful and healing spark of life calling from beneath the years and layers of your eating disorder.

Ask yourself: What is your eating disorder doing for you? Why is it necessary for that healing spark to work so hard to call out to you and be heard?

You may be using your eating disorder to keep yourself from knowing just how bad you believe life can get. You may be afraid to let people in your life know what you are going through and what you really want. So part of your eating disorder exists to keep the peace. It dulls you down so you are in a state of acceptance of the unacceptable. People close to you believe you accept your way of life. In fact, you are (or were) resigned to live with an eating disorder that prevents you from becoming aware of more possibilities. You have been blocking what you fear to know in order to maintain peace in your life.

It may be against the law of the land to disturb the peace, but it's not against the law to speak your truth and pursue your happiness. So here is where you begin. You need to know where you are standing before you can take your first step.

Vanessa, thirty-seven and recently divorced, sat alone at the kitchen table in her temporary rented house, in emotional pain and with no direction. She had two teenage sons and was suffering from bulimia and anorexia alternately. Vanessa, trembling and blinking through tears, tried to help herself by making a list. It was a list of her feelings, her actions, and what her life looked like. She tried to clear her mind of despair so she could look at herself from an objective point of view. She wanted to address each item as if it were a task to complete.

Here is a list of her entries. They may apply to you, too. Use it and elaborate on it to make the list fully your own. You are not alone. Others have been where you are and have moved through to recovery. Listen to the voice of your pain and the voice of the hopeful healing spark that guides you.

Vanessa began her list with one question, "What makes me miserable about being me?"

1. Poor health (this includes effect on teeth, bones, and menses)
2. Shame
3. Loneliness
4. Outbreaks of rage
5. Losing track of time in chunks or small blips
6. Crying jags
7. Morning anxiety
8. Needing to lie to people
9. Shoplifting? Food, certainly. Other things — books, jewelry once, and napkins and spoons from restaurants
10. Bouts of despair
11. Being fat
12. Not being able to start building a better life

Your list can stand as a baseline for you that can remind you of your recovery progress.

Memory is quirky when you have an eating disorder. Some experiences fade because you don't give them attention. Some fade because you are in denial or too anxious to focus. And sometimes, for reasons we may never know, you gradually might slide back into acting out your eating disorder.

When this happens, and it happens to everyone, the list you are making now will still exist. Even if you destroy it, you could buy this book again and turn to this chapter. Your beginning place is solid. You can use what you create here as a starting point for recovery practices and as a safety net to catch you when you fall. More than that, you can use it as a friendly and familiar place to grab hold, get back on your path, learn and continue.

You may not appreciate yet how the items on your list relate to your eating disorder. You may think that your troubles of undereating or overeating and all the behaviors that go with it (like purging, hiding food, bingeing in secret, etc.) are the full extent of your eating disorder and that your task is to stop doing these things.

You might believe there's an upside to

your eating disorder behaviors because sometimes you look forward to a binge or hours on the treadmill. Yet, when you see how your eating disorder is related to the behaviors and feelings on your list, any imagined benefits fall apart.

Look at the conflict between what you want out of life versus what is required to maintain your eating disorder. You want genuine companionship, praise, love, and respect from people, but you have to keep your true self and current way of living hidden. You use some of your eating disorder behaviors to give you the "look" you believe you need for companionship, but you continue to find fault with your appearance. You want to control other people's perception so they see an image of you that is perfection and not you as you perceive yourself. Yet you feel lonely when you can't share your genuine experience. You want to feel safe and relaxed, yet you live under the stress of anticipating that you could be discovered as a fake at any time. This is an exhausting way to live.

Yet, in the secret world you create with your eating disorder, you do find some pleasure and relaxation. You feel confident and competent when you arrange for privacy in just the right setting with all your favorite binge foods. It can be fun to put on your loose-fitting clothes and select TV shows or several DVDs to get you through your binge. You've given yourself hours of unscheduled time for your big date with yourself — a total binge-fest. No one is home to interrupt your bingeing. You can throw up as many times as you like without having to hide the sound by running water in the tap or shower.

Instead of a binge-fest, you might have a date with the treadmill and run, even through agonizing pain. These planned episodes may bring you relief from anxiety for a while. You have a feeling of accomplishment because you created the time, space, and items you need for your binge/purge or treadmill episode. But doesn't desperation come in quickly? Aren't you frightened when the movie or program ends and you are in the real world again, surrounded by litter from your binge, your bloated belly aching, worried that you might not be able to throw it all up, scared that someone might come home early?

Your eating disorder seems to promise to get you through the day, the night, or the weekend by taking you to emotional peace. It assures you that you'll be safe, beautiful, protected, and able to hide what you want to. It swears that it will soothe and comfort you, promises that you can stay on task when you are anxious. Further, it promises that you don't need anybody or anything as long as you have your eating disorder by your side. You are willing and eager to leave the reality of your life based on those promises. But does your eating disorder deliver on these promises in reality? Can you see how your eating disorder actually perpetuates your isolation and loneliness?

The beauty promise is something to explore. You can't identify someone with an eating disorder by looking at her body. Someone suffering from an eating disorder might be obese, moderately heavy, a healthy weight, moderately thin, or emaciated. Someone at all levels of weight, including obese and emaciated, may *not* have an eating disorder.

If you are striving for the body beautiful, is it your goal to be able to look great for an occasion or to look great as you go about your normal activities? Do you need to apply cold water or ice on your neck glands, swollen from purging, to look good? Do you wear makeup to hide your haggardness and poor skin tone from starving? What physical consequences does your eating disorder deliver? Is it making you beautiful if you

78

have to pour money into dentistry, plastic surgery, orthopedists, and nutritionists? What would it take for you to rebel against this giver of false promises?

When you recognize the false promises coming from your eating disorder, you are getting ready to recognize false promises coming from people in your life and from our culture as well. Paying attention to the lies your eating disorder tells is the first step in freeing you from the yoke of false promises so you can build a substantial life in reality.

You cannot identify the hypocrisy and false promises your eating disorder offers if you continue to defend your actions. When you believe false promises, you keep your disorder a secret, deny its control over you, and, when confronted, protest that the concern is not justified. Your life is fine, you are in control, and you can stop any time you want and others should mind their own business.

You don't want to recognize the extent that lies and false promises cripple your life. If you did, you could be overwhelmed by debilitating shame. You've lost weight and regained. You've gained weight and lost it again. You've weaned yourself off the treadmill once, but now you're running yourself to the bone again. You're isolated because you know people will see your body and wonder what has happened to you.

As you approach your genuine torment, you approach your genuine recovery work. . . . You are afraid you will pass your eating disorder on to your children. You are weary of looking into the toilet bowl while you are retching. You want to stop worrying about breaking your bones, hurting your heart, ravaging your esophagus, and destroying your teeth. You want to stop having an eating disorder.

Stop. Breathe. Instead of focusing on what you want to stop, focus on what you want to start. Ask yourself, "What could my life look like if I were free of this eating disorder?" Below is a list of possibilities. Check off what applies to you and add more that come to your heart and mind.

WHAT COULD MY LIFE LOOK LIKE IF I WERE FREE OF THIS EATING DISORDER?

1. I have no secrets.
2. I don't lie.
3. I'm at ease around food.
4. I say what I think.
5. I form friendships based on mutual respect.

6. I am confident and generous.
7. I let people see the real me.
8. I love sincerely.
9. I allow and accept love from other people.

With your eating disorder gone, ask: "What happens to my health?" You may not know specifically how your eating disorder affects your body and mind, but you know it must. A beginning list of possibilities could be:

How could my health improve if I didn't have an eating disorder anymore?

1. I think more clearly.
2. I have more physical energy.
3. I menstruate on a regular basis.
4. My teeth and gums are healthy.
5. My heart and digestive system function with less stress.

As you recover you will experience unexpected joy as your body reveals to you the benefits of living in health. Your physical symptoms come from malnutrition, excessive exercise, sleep deprivation, and lack of basic self-care plus the stress of maintaining your eating disorder. When this stress ends in recovery, you will find yourself more at ease with other people and in your own skin.

These may sound like false promises to you. Living with an eating disorder, you are accustomed to false promises. But, in time, you'll discover these benefits for yourself.

In the present, as you read these pages, your eating disordered mind asks, "What will people think if I don't have my eating disorder, and they see me for what and who I am?" With that thought, the fears and fantasies that power your eating disorder rise up in a torrent of self-condemnations: "I am unlovable, ugly, stupid, boring, incompetent, inadequate, and unacceptable in all ways. Don't try to trick me with health. Health means being fat."

You may be shaking your head at this and asking "How can I know that these harsh judgments are not true?" I know they are untrue because you have an eating disorder, and I also had one.

Look at what you've been doing to figure out and carry out the necessary activities for getting your binge foods, keeping your activities secret, having a private place to act out, gathering the financial resources to get your supplies, and creating appropriate and convincing lies when necessary. These are skills and talents that, unfortunately, you use against yourself. However, they are your natural resources, and you can use them for something else once you no longer need your eating disorder. That's how I know.

Let your wise voice support you as you twist and turn your way through these fears. They are barriers that will keep you stuck in your eating disorder. It's time to come out and become the healthy, vibrant woman you are meant to be.

You will find exercises and activities in Appendix B that will help you confront and eradicate the false and harsh criticisms you have for yourself.

I remember visiting my friend Ingeborg one afternoon. She was in her late seventies. Ingeborg was a modest woman with a brilliant and tenacious mind. She translated psychology textbooks from English into Swedish. She was also a gourmet cook, and she created a warm and loving home not only for her family but for those of us fortunate enough to be invited in. I knew she practiced yoga every morning with a program on television and had been doing so for many years. She didn't talk about her yoga just as she didn't talk about her many considerable achievements.

On this particular visit, I watched her

preparing our meal. This was always a pleasure. I saw her move rapidly along the side of the kitchen counter holding a heavy bowl and spatula. A low cupboard door was open, and she gracefully extended her left foot to close the door without spilling anything from the bowl or losing momentum on her way to the stove. It was an elegant and highly functional move.

I said, "Ah. I see your yoga." She didn't understand me at first, because the move was so natural and spontaneous to her. Yet she did agree that without a daily yoga practice she might not have been able to do it.

The exercises and activities in this book are like her yoga. As you practice, your way of thinking, perceiving, and experiencing the world will deepen and expand. You will naturally respond to your challenges in a more graceful and productive way.

I offer you a new exercise — backtracking — to do at least once a week in addition to breathing, affirmations, and journaling. Backtracking stretches your mind and awareness. It's also helpful in grounding yourself when you need to make a decision.

BACKTRACKING

Pick an item of food. Trace it back to where it began. Go back as far as you can, paying attention to the hands, minds, hearts, and backs of the people who were involved in the chain that brought it to your table.

For example, consider an apple. Take it from your hand to your refrigerator, to the grocery bag you carried it in to your car, to the market display, to the storage bin, to the truck, the loading dock, and all the people who picked and packed the apple, to the farmers who planted the seeds. See if you can get to the orchard and the individual tree.

You can do this with any item of food. You eventually can do this with anything at all as a mind-expanding and even soul-expanding exercise. Your goal is to make your presence more real in the world. Part of that involves making your food and the forces that brought your food to your hands more real to you. You can then appreciate foods that nourish your mind, body, and spirit. You can share food with someone else in the spirit of nourishing their minds, bodies, and spirits. Plus, you will feel connected with the energies of countless people who provide us all with our food. This is the beginning of the end of your isolation.

In recovery, food stops being an object of instant gratification, just as you stop being an object and become the authentic woman you are.

You are developing the inner resources you need to cope with your emerging feelings without using food to numb yourself. As you develop your new strengths and inner resilience, you will be able to tolerate your healing experiences, and you will need your eating disorder less.

DAILY EXERCISES

1. Follow your breath for five minutes at least three times a day.
2. Read or recite your three affirmations twenty times each at least three times a day. See Appendix A, "Affirmations."
3. Write freely on any of the questions in this chapter or any items from your lists.
4. Each day this week, pick a food item and backtrack with it. If you are feeling particularly daring, try backtracking with a binge food item.

CHAPTER 5
BOUNDARIES: A CHALLENGE IN EARLY RECOVERY

"We do not act rightly because we have virtue or excellence, but we rather have those because we have acted rightly."
— Aristotle

The foremost eating disorder recovery issue, from my experience, is learning to recognize and honor boundaries. Once you respect and set essential boundaries, you can develop vital recovery tools. This is the critical work that allows you to say no or yes in a way that is meaningful and honest.

When I was in my first trembling stages of recovery, I remember my therapist telling me that unless I could choose to say no, my yes was meaningless. This was a revelation to me. I, like most people with eating disorders, had little understanding of the concept of boundaries. I believed that my people-pleasing yes would get me through most situations and that my no would cause others to be angry and reject me.

Being unaware of boundaries creates havoc in your life. You are bewildered by another person's response (or lack of response) to you because you crossed a boundary you didn't know was there. When you can't identify or respect your own boundaries, it's unlikely that you recognize or respect the boundaries of others.

Right now, you don't know about limits or the experience of "enough," relating to food. But you also don't recognize cues in the world that signal you to slow down or stop. Because of this, you can lose friends, career opportunities, and social connections without knowing why. You can attract unsavory people, even those you find abhorrent, because you said or otherwise implied yes to ease yourself through a situation rather than saying a sincere no.

Throughout the exercises and activities in this book, you will be working on boundary recognition and the inner strength you need to set limits. The tasks are simple, and you can do them throughout the day at almost any time to help you build boundary awareness.

BOUNDARY RECOGNITION

Boundaries are limits. They mark a separation between what's mine and what's yours, this and that, that and that, you and me, one person and another. Boundaries are lines between legal and illegal, healthy and unhealthy, safe and unsafe, private and public, sacred and profane. Boundaries are lines between too much and enough and between too little and enough. Boundaries are lines between what's fair and unfair. They define countries, cities, private and public properties, jobs, status, relationships, and the roles we play in our families and communities.

Visible boundaries are fences, doors, gates, roads, sidewalks, railroad tracks, signs, windows, and bars. Invisible boundaries are clear when a barking or growling dog warns that you are encroaching upon his acceptable limits. He may defend his boundary if you cross it. A person may look uncomfortable and step back or ask you to step back if you have come too close to his or her spatial boundary.

Acceptable boundaries differ across cultures and time. Whether consciously recognized or not, boundaries maintain a desired status quo in human functioning, and when you cross a boundary, you disrupt the status quo. The impact of the disruption determines the consequence. Boundaries can be negotiated and adjusted, but they can't be ignored without consequence.

My ex-husband was in the Air Force, and as a second lieutenant and officer of the day on a small airbase he fielded phone calls that reported problems. On weekends the calls were few and usually not too serious, such as drunken airmen crashing into the base gate. When my husband was a captain on a much larger base, the first call he got as officer of the day was about a border incident in the Middle East. He was shocked at the magnitude of the change but realized that all boundary incidents were *border incidents.*

What is the nature of the border incidents in your daily life? Your body needs a certain amount of nourishment to live. That amount is finite. Your eating choices reflect your acknowledgment of that boundary. Too much or too little create border incidents with consequences to your health.

To maintain your lifestyle, you need a certain amount of financing. Budgets are a collection of small boundaries making up a defined allocation of funds. Disregarding those boundaries will have consequences for your lifestyle.

Boundaries are inextricably connected to the source of authority. To develop and maintain a relationship, you need to respect your boundaries and the boundaries of the other person. What's his is his, and what's yours is yours. This includes possessions, time, money, expertise, connections, relationships, even personal energy. You can give because you are the authority of yours. You cannot take. His can come to you only through gifts or permission.

When you cross someone's boundary, you defy their authority. When someone crosses your boundary, they defy your authority. Unauthorized boundary crossing brings up powerful emotions with concrete consequences. Here are some examples of boundary crossings that can create border incidents.

Susan takes clothes from her sister's closet and lipstick from her purse without asking. She also commits her sister to projects without checking first.

Mary, waiting for her friend while she dresses, uses her friend's computer without asking. At a party, she rummages through the hostess's kitchen cupboards and the medicine cabinet. These are violations of boundaries.

Taking a book off someone's bookshelf in

a public area of their home is not a boundary crossing. The shelf, placed in a public place, is a tacit statement of permission to use. But when Susan and Mary assume an authority that is not theirs, they've disregarded a boundary and can harm a relationship.

When you give permission for someone to cross your boundary, you authorize them to move through a barrier. You give a friend or employee the keys to your home. You give your webmaster certain passwords. You allow a family member to call you at work.

Your ability to say no is critical. If you agree to a boundary crossing because you want to please someone, you are crossing your own boundaries. For example, you may let someone borrow your car even if you know they are accident prone, or loan money to someone who is financially irresponsible. You may work longer hours for no pay or lend your talents to someone else's project at the cost of neglecting your own projects out of a need to be liked.

If you have an eating disorder, you don't honor boundaries associated with food. You eat too much or too little. You say, "This is the last time," regularly. This means, "This is the last time I will cross this boundary," and not binge or throw up or steal food.

Because you can't keep your promises to yourself, you become casual with limits. You develop a habit of accepting unauthorized boundary crossings. Worse, you feel powerless to stop someone from invading your boundaries. What you say to yourself about crossing boundaries with your eating disorder you will repeat in other boundary crossing situations: "One more time and then I'm done . . . This is a special circumstance . . . I'm special and can get away with it this one time . . ."

A person crossing your boundaries will justify their actions. They might say, "I didn't think you would mind. I needed something to wear and you weren't here." The person feels that defying your authority is fine. "But I'm your _____ (fill in the blank: mother, friend, employer, partner, neighbor, child)." In other words, the person feels entitled to what is yours. In your people-pleasing mode you may allow this person to violate your authority and could harbor a resentment that will trigger your eating disorder.

Passive energy can become active or explosive at a boundary. This is where the expression, "Good fences make good neighbors" comes from. The limitation defines territory and keeps the peace.

But what if you meet a boundary you don't like and don't want to accept? A simple story goes like this: Elsa is working on an important project when her printer runs out of ink. She's out of spares, and she needs a new cartridge so she can meet her deadline. It's early evening. She drives to her local computer store and arrives just as it is closing. The sign on the door reads "Closed." The lights are still on, and she sees people inside. Elsa knocks on the door. No one pays attention. She bangs on the door. Someone looks her way. She says, "Please let me in." The man shakes his head and points to his watch. She's frustrated and tries to show her need.

"Please," she says. "It will only take a minute." In that request Elsa is asking the employee to let her cross his time boundary. She says, "This is a special circumstance. It's for my special project — just one time." She is asking him to make her concerns and her time more important than his.

Elsa, like many people who don't recognize boundaries, has a sense of entitlement. She thinks to herself and sometimes actually says, "But this is *me*. It's okay because it's *me*. I need more than you do. I'll use it better than you will."

Unauthorized boundary crossings hurt relationships, marriages, businesses, and international peace. They cause lawsuits, criminal proceedings, divorce, and job loss. They also contribute to keeping your eating disorder powerful and tenacious.

Disregarding boundaries is not a fundamental aspect of your personality. It is a developmental issue. Elsa's eating disorder kept her from developing respect for how boundaries create safety and make relationships possible. She will override a boundary she doesn't see because she is trying to get what she needs, in the same way that she will eat more than her body can tolerate because she needs the food to quell her anxiety.

If you binge, you must go full speed ahead, filling yourself up with food or merchandise or activity. You try to endlessly fill yourself so you have no room for a thought or insight that might disturb your protective system and illusion of safety.

If you suffer from anorexia, you do the same thing in reverse. Your restriction is endless. You don't eat enough nourishment to sustain a healthy body. You live a life that is noticeable by its sparseness. You allow yourself less than the minimum in safety, intimate relationships, and self care. Using a lowercase "i" to identify yourself feels right to you. On occasion, you become frantic and plead or demand help from others only to refuse help that's offered.

When you don't recognize the natural limits of your body, you can wind up in the hospital after starving too thoroughly and then bingeing out of control. Your body can't handle the extremes. You spontaneously throw up food and blood and pass out. Your own body and gravity stop you. When you can't set and honor boundaries, you are at the mercy of natural limits you can't control. At the tragic extreme, endlessly losing or gaining weight ends with death.

With no personal sense of healthy boundaries, you have no concept or inclination to eat when you haven't eaten enough or to stop eating when you have.

Just as the woman who compulsively eats and wants to return to endless filling, you want to return to endless deprivation. That's where you feel you are in control and have a chance to be safe. How frustrating it is for the anorexic woman to reach size zero and have no place to go. Clothes sizes don't go into negative numbers.

How can you stop yourself from your eating disorder actions if you can't place limits on your behavior? You've had what you consider past successes when you did stop because of a diet program, but you lost control and reverted to your old ways, often gaining more weight or losing more weight than before the diet. You couldn't keep to the structure on a permanent basis. Your eating disorder crashed through limits and took charge.

Once you recognize, respect, and honor limits and boundaries, you can make great strides in your recovery. Your recovery is not about using willpower to stop destructive behavior or start healthier behavior and reasonable eating habits. Your recovery is about developing beyond your current limitations.

It takes many small steps to establish healthy boundaries you can honor and maintain. Learning to appreciate "enough" is part of your challenge. "Not enough" is the same as "too much" in the following exercises. As you strive to reach enough, be wary of reaching for perfection. The line that separates enough from too much or too little can be substantial and represents more of a range than a razor's edge.

In the following areas — sleep, food, and friends — find a range between too little and too much that works for you.

Establish a reasonable bedtime and wakeup time that works for your life. Make sure you get eight hours of sleep each night. Work up to the eight hours gradually, if necessary. Adjust your activities so that you are in bed in time to get those hours.

Sleep deprivation is associated with many serious consequences to your well-being, including: heart attack and heart failure, stroke, obesity, depression, attention deficit disorder (ADD) mental impairment, fetal and childhood growth retardation and injury from accidents. It also reinforces and intensifies your eating disorder symptoms. You may learn that some problems you thought you had to live with forever clear up once you give yourself adequate, nourishing sleep.

Give yourself a few months to find your best sleep routine. You know what too little sleep means for you. But too much sleep can lull your mind and contribute to isolation. Eventually you might find that you do well on seven and a half or eight and a half or nine hours. See how it goes. Your body may need months to make up for deprivation or chaotic patterns before you can adjust to getting enough sleep on a regular basis. Be patient with yourself.

FOOD

Decide what you need before you go grocery shopping. You can make adjustments at the store, but stay close to your original plan. As you make your shopping list, take into consideration your healthy eating plans for the day or week. Make adjustments in the store in terms of substitutions. For example, substitute tuna for salmon or spinach for broccoli, but not cookies for oranges. Keep to the amounts that you originally planned. See how you feel when you honor the limits you've established.

One way to establish limits when eating at home is to serve yourself food on pretty plates that are the right size for adequate portions.

FRIENDS

Be clear to yourself about your time and schedule when you make arrangements to get together with a friend. Think about your commitments before and after the meeting, so you can not only be on time, but have enough time for your friend.

Find out what your friend's personal preferences are in terms of phone calls and honor those boundaries. Issues might include calls during dinner time, calls after 9:00 p.m. or before 9:00 a.m., calls at work, or calls during their children's bath and bedtime, or on weekends. Consider time limits for phone conversations, too, by establishing time boundaries in advance. Keep phone calls short, or ask if your friend has time to speak longer. Ask, "Is this a good time?" If it isn't, ask when a good time to catch up might be. When visiting, respect the agreed upon arrival time and establish when it's time for you to leave.

Sometimes these agreed upon boundaries can crash into your emotional needs. You may be feeling anxious or sad or lonely and crave emotional support. This is part of your eating disorder recovery challenge. You honor your friend's boundaries and take only what your friend can give. If you are left unsatisfied and emotionally raw, seek additional support elsewhere, while you continue to honor boundaries.

Here's an example of a boundary misunderstanding that may be familiar to you from either side of the relationship. Susan feels like she's found a great friend whom she can visit and spend all night talking with. To her, it's a bonding experience. Susan doesn't understand why her great new friend doesn't call after their first meeting.

If you have an eating disorder, you may

misinterpret or simply not see cues people give you. These cues, including both words and body language, signal boundary information. If you do notice, you may push for a little more time or attention the same way you rationalize and push for another box of cookies or another twenty minutes on the treadmill.

Susan didn't realize she had "binged" on her hostess, who didn't appreciate that she crossed an energy and time limit. Her hostess may have difficulty in setting boundaries, too. She didn't say, "I need to stop talking and go to bed now." Or "My children need me to get up early with them." Susan's hostess couldn't find a way to say, "We have to draw this evening to a close." Or maybe she did, and her efforts were feeble in an attempt to be polite and inoffensive. Or maybe her efforts were straightforward, but Susan disregarded them or didn't recognize them as cues. Susan may be disappointed and bewildered that her new friend hasn't called. She doesn't realize that because she could not recognize her friend's discomfort signals or appreciate her limits, her friend is reluctant to spend more time with her. Her friend can't afford endless conversations.

Another variation on boundary oblivion is the continual helper. Letisha offers to help her friends by caring for their animals or their children, house-sitting while they are away, helping them prepare for parties, or cleaning up afterwards. She will listen to actors read their lines. She will help her friend do accounting for his new business. Letisha is thoughtful and thoroughly generous. She gives more than she can afford. She leaves little time, energy, or money for herself. Her life suffers from lack of attention.

If this seems like your life, you may not notice that others can be overwhelmed by your generosity and may be uncomfortable because they know they could never reciprocate at the same level. Alternatively, some people will be glad to take what is offered so freely and consider you a reliable resource who never requires payment. They may feel sorry for you because, with all your giving, you seem needy and desperate for involvement. They may feel charitable toward you and give you tasks so you don't feel alone, or they may feel superior to you and experiment with just how far they can go in taking advantage of you. All these examples reveal a lack of authority in the helper about establishing and enforcing personal boundaries.

If you don't see boundaries and can't set limits, you will give too much and take too much. You will feel drained because you use your time and energy for others while your own life wilts. You will feel neglected by the people in your life and taken for granted. You will seethe with resentment. If you have an eating disorder, you will eat or starve to soothe your emotional pain and to cover your resentment, and you won't know why.

Once you appreciate that recognizing and respecting boundaries brings more quality to your life, you can use your eating disorder behavior as a guide and teacher. When you reach for your eating disorder, ask yourself, "Is there a boundary violation going on somewhere in my life?" You can experiment and practice setting healthy boundaries in eating as preparation and training for setting healthy boundaries in all areas of your life.

Your goal is to mindfully explore your behavior to discover your necessary boundaries. Rather than follow strict rules dictated by a program or yourself, go on an exploratory adventure to discover the meaning of "enough." On this adventure of discovery you gradually learn to eat not-too-much and not-too-little. You eat healthful, non-toxic foods that nourish your body. You discover the timing that is right for you, usually meaning that you eat every day and not less often than every four hours.

Along with food boundaries, you honor other boundaries to give your body essential nourishment. To be well hydrated without creating water toxicity, you need to drink six to eight glasses of plain water a day — not less and not more. You give yourself approximately eight hours sleep a night. You do some kind of aerobic exercise for thirty minutes to an hour a day at least three days a week.

This may seem a stretch from where you are now. It may seem boring, or unreachable. It may seem that on such a plan you would become fat. It may seem like pure fantasy and impossible. Yet, to be healthy and well, this is basic health maintenance for human beings. When you no longer live by your eating disorder patterns, this is the healthy way you live.

As you search for the meaning of enough, you may need to call a supportive friend to let them know you're committing to a daily eating, sleeping, or exercise schedule. Checking in with a friend on your progress helps you continue your search for the meaning of "enough." Once the sense of what is sufficient for your needs is your own, you will recognize your mind and body cues and honor signals that tell you when you need more or less or when you have achieved that magic amount: enough. The skills it takes to recognize what signals enough for you will heighten your awareness of boundaries and limits for other situations as well.

To get there from here is an emotional journey that does not begin with food. You start by building your capacity to emotionally tolerate the changes that are coming. Now is your time to develop ways to encourage, support, and sustain you as you develop and recognize healthy boundaries for eating and for living your life.

Here are some suggestions to develop more authority in setting and honoring time boundaries. As a general practice, schedule your week. Write down your obligations as well as your appointments. Allow for specific amounts of time to do your tasks and spell that out in your appointment notebook. Do your best to honor your self-imposed commitments.

To practice time management, do the following half-hour exercise. Get a timer, some paper, crayons, a pen, glue, scissors, and a packet of colorful stickers. You'll be completing small tasks in five-minute rounds.

Round 1: Color a sheet of paper in

whatever way you like, but stop immediately at five minutes.

Round 2: Cut out shapes. Stop after five minutes.

Round 3: Decorate the shapes. Stop after five minutes.

Round 4: Glue your cutouts to the paper. Stop after five minutes.

Round 5: Add stickers wherever you like for five minutes only.

Round 6: You now have five more minutes to complete your project using any of the materials you wish. Again, you must stop after five minutes.

This exercise gives you a sense of how much you can accomplish when you plan your actions and honor boundaries. It teaches your mind how to function within boundaries. You will be challenged when you want to do less or more in an interval. Yet this exercise can be a pleasant way to soothe and reassure yourself when you are stressed while simultaneously strengthening your respect for boundaries.

You can adapt this half-hour exercise to any series of small tasks. For example, you can clean a room by doing a series of five-minute tasks. Set your time for five minutes each and stop on time.

1. Sort clutter
2. Remove trash
3. Dust furniture
4. Sweep the floor

Here's another. Sit at your computer and complete this series of five-minute tasks:

1. Check e-mail
2. Respond to e-mails
3. Check social media sites
4. Respond where appropriate

These exercises do not take the place of long tasks. They serve to remind you that you can set boundaries and do more than you think you can in short bursts. Plus, these exercises serve to give you a break from a long task and move you into something you've neglected because you believed you didn't have time for it.

Scheduling yourself like this strengthens your ability to say no because accepting an interruption will disrupt your exercise. You will learn to say, "I'll get back to you." You will also learn to not answer the phone sometimes or to resist responding immediately to your e-mail. This strengthens your ability to postpone gratification. You start developing the awareness muscles that will serve you well in your life and self-care.

If you start judging yourself, criticizing yourself, or punishing yourself for not doing a boundary exercise perfectly, please know that this harshness is a symptom of your eating disorder. The treasure lies in unearthing what those boundary breakdowns are really about — where you leave a structure and surrender your own authority. What is going for you in that moment? What does your boundary crossing accomplish for you? Is it worth it to you?

Recognizing and honoring boundaries of any kind is a challenge for someone with an eating disorder. Here are some simple legal limits to explore at this stage. This quiz will help you discover areas where you can practice honoring limits.

DO YOU . . .
- cross at cross walks?
- stop at stop signs and stoplights?
- buckle up?
- cross with the light?
- signal when making a turn?

- shoplift?
- eat food at a grocery store without paying?
- return library books?
- return objects you've borrowed?

Remember, these exercises are not created in order to judge you or to punish you. To establish solid recovery, you need to look at what is actually going on in your life. Any kind of boundary violation relates to your recovery. Set limits for yourself where you can. Do not "binge" on the exercises.

Keep track of your illegal boundary crossings. Over time, you will gain insight into what these crossings mean to you and why you do it. For example, if you steal, you may want the feelings associated with what you took, rather than the item itself. If you can afford to buy the item, why would you steal it? Did you feel you had to steal time or attention from an important person to feel comforted and nourished as you were or wished you were when you were a child?

You may steal an item like a piece of jewelry from someone because you want to possess a quality of that person. You don't know yet how to give yourself openly what you need. Look to your secret desires. If you have to hide what matters to you, even from yourself, you will snatch at false substitutes, even when that means stealing. Part of recovery is knowing what you genuinely want in life and learning how to create a way to give it to yourself while respecting boundaries.

When you have an eating disorder, you can feel inadequate and inferior. Periodically, a situation will present itself where you can compensate by defying your beliefs about yourself. You switch to suddenly taking a position of superiority. For a moment, or more, you place yourself above the law. You don't stop at a stop sign. You disregard the speed limit. You believe laws don't apply to you. These also may be the beliefs you have when you are eating more or less than is good for you.

Journal about your illegal boundary crossing. As you write, include what was going on in your life at the time and how you felt in the moment. You will be learning and gaining strength and appreciation for what you need but had no way to give yourself until now.

If you don't recognize or understand boundaries between people, it may be that you never had an opportunity to learn about them. If you didn't experience a reliable source of protection and safety when you were young and helpless, you may not have experienced an awareness of boundaries. Your state of existential aloneness can feel as if you are lost in limitless space and falling all the time. Bingeing, stealing, grabbing hold of anything that gives you a sense of safety becomes your way of getting relief from that endless fall. Hurtling along the highway, enjoying the rush and not feeling restrained by speed limits gives you, with your lack of boundaries, relief and takes you to an elated state where, instead of feeling powerless, you feel powerful. You can get a similar feeling when you disregard social limits. You may interrupt others to take the limelight, flirt with a married man, or sit in a chair of authority that is not yours. Stealing is part of an impulsive rush toward relief.

When the essence of a child's forming identity is ignored or purposefully, or through ignorance, disrespected, the child learns that pain or bewilderment is her natural state. If her personal boundaries are not respected, she doesn't learn to recognize or respect the boundaries of others. A child has nothing to compare with her experience. Everything is happening to her for the first time and informs her of what to expect from the world. If a girl is physically or sexually abused, the abuser ignores the integrity of her person and her spirit. If this happens regularly and is accepted by care-takers, the girl lives in fear that she can be attacked at any time. She has no respected boundary that keeps an abuser at bay. She also learns to hide from other people, please them, or lash out at them in an attempt to protect herself, even if she is with people who do respect her. Moreover, if a child is regularly exposed to violence, even if it's not directed at her, she will do her best to escape into a private world to give herself a sense of safety in fantasy. She learns to go blank or numb to avoid the ugly stress around her. She has no boundaries to protect her except the internal force she uses to shut down her awareness.

Boundary invasion can occur in more subtle ways, like overwhelming a child with too much stimulation and gifts, or taking objects or activities away from a child regularly for reasons the child cannot understand. The child sees no criteria for behavior or for her gains or losses.

If a child receives conflicting messages from her caretakers, she learns that what people say is not reliable. "Yes, you can have that dress, but we can't tell your father." "Yes, you can have that drink, but don't tell anyone." Or, "George is cheating on his wife, but don't tell anyone." Or, "I'll do your homework for you, if you write your brother's paper. The teacher doesn't have to know." Such messages show her that she has the right to disrespect boundaries, while simultaneously creating mistrust as she learns that others will disregard her in the same way.

More bewilderment about boundaries develops when a child discovers her possessions are missing because the prevailing family assumption is that anyone can take anything from anyone at any time and nothing is private.

Any one of these examples, lived on a routine basis early in life, prevents a child from developing a sense of boundaries. Such a lack contributes to naïve boundary crossings and an underlying experience of nameless anxiety.

As you proceed with these exercises you may have personal revelations about how your boundaries were invaded. Situations and memories may come up in your journaling. As you experience anger or disappointment or grief, do your breathing exercise, affirmations, and journaling to help you tolerate and clear these feelings from your system. This is important work that must not be minimized. You need to be conscientious.

Boundaries also relate to personal space. Every human senses what kind of space they need around them. If someone steps into your space, you will feel the shift in the dynamic of the relationship. If a man comes too close, you may feel threatened. On the other hand, you may feel self-conscious and acutely aware of him because you experience the boundary crossing as intimate, perhaps with romantic or sexual connotations.

You may feel disgusted because an unappealing woman or man presses against you. You may feel delighted and relieved of tension at a formal dinner when the host's children cross their time and space boundaries and enter the room pajama clad pleading for a glass of water or a hug. You may feel embarrassed for the same reason.

You can get an indication of your own personal space by paying attention when you walk on a public sidewalk and see a person walking toward you. At a certain distance, you can look at her. You can watch her mannerisms, her clothes, and her facial expressions. As you approach one another, however, you drop your eyes. She's too close now for that kind of observation. You may feel uncomfortable that she will be looking at you too closely.

If you don't stop observing her, you run the risk of violating the boundary that defines her personal space. You will notice that she drops her eyes or gives you a look that lets you know you are now in her personal territory. She may frown or look nervous. She may greet you as a friend she thinks she's forgotten. She may grimace or glare at you to warn you off.

By being alert in this way, you learn where your personal line is and discover responses from others when their personal space is violated. This is practice to help you be aware of your own personal space and recognize signals others give you about theirs. For example, if a woman ignores or is unaware of a physical spatial boundary between herself and a man, and if she crosses over into his space, she may be surprised that he considers her action a sexual invitation.

These examples are the nonverbal and ever-present boundary challenges all of us face every day. When is overhearing a conversation acceptable, and when is it eavesdropping? When is making a sugges-tion to someone about their clothing or home acceptable conversation, and when is it presumptuous and offensive? Recognizing boundaries is essential for all of us.

Human beings also have boundaries regarding health and beauty maintenance. These are principles that govern self-care behavior. How often and how much do you need to eat, sleep, drink water, exercise, bathe, and clean your environment? If you don't have a natural feel for what is too much or not enough, you need to think each self-care item through methodically.

As you develop and heal, you will be able to reflect on your feelings and determine what and how much self-care and self-nourishment you need. For example, bodies require nourishment to repair, sustain, and function, and you need a certain proportion and variety of foods to meet those requirements. I write this in as formal and objective a way as I can. The word "diet" looms in the back of your mind like a threat and a reminder of failures. I am not talking about a weight gain, weight loss or maintenance diet. I am talking about the reality of what kind of fuel your vehicle needs to run well, and how often you need to fill your tank.

Food and eating are emotionally-loaded topics. Body appearance, aging, levels of beauty, weight, skin tone, muscle tone, quality and amount of hair, and the texture of your nails can be emotionally-loaded topics. When you strip the emotional load from physical care, you are left with the boundaries of nature. If you cross those boundaries, you will experience consequences. Much of the dieting and weight loss or weight gain industry is dedicated to bypassing natural consequences. Such diet programs promise quick weight change and a happier life but don't tell you about the serious health risks associated with quick weight gain or loss. The false promises feed into your unhappiness and desire for fast relief. It's difficult for the weight loss industry to attract customers and make money by selling you an unglamorous and gradual way to develop health, strength, and confidence so you live at the healthy weight that is right for you.

Ask yourself, "How do I cross boundaries with food and bypass natural consequences?" The answer to that question is the heart of eating disorder behavior. Eat a lot but avoid the calories by throwing up; eat normally but run off the calories or starve every other day; eat but have surgery to remove fat; binge but isolate so no one sees you; don't eat but get implants in order to fake healthy volume where you want it. The list goes on. Whether you eat too much or starve, you can attempt to hide consequences by wearing loose-fitting clothes and touch up photographs so you project an appearance you don't really have.

I remember visiting Louise, a forty-five-year-old woman in the hospital. She qualified for the EDNO diagnosis. Louise was recovering from a near fatal heart attack and had lost massive amounts of weight. She had in the past undergone cheek, breast, and buttocks implant surgeries, face lifts, and facial sculpturing. When I saw her, she was like a pale, fragile stick of a woman. She said, "I'm glad I had the implants. They are the only part of me that looks substantial now."

We'll address the food-related boundary issues in another chapter. Right now our goal is to build your awareness and appreciation for boundaries in general. With a greater sense of awareness, you will be able to adjust your methods of approaching boundaries — yours as well as other people's — with wisdom and confidence while being mindful of your own self-care.

For example, if your mother or mother-in-law questions your taste in furniture, clothes, or books, do you challenge her if you disagree? Or do you contain your feelings in silence and alter your behavior to suit her? Do you have authority in your home? Do you collapse your boundaries and surrender under criticism, pressure, or even mild comments?

Increasing your awareness of your attitudes and habits regarding boundaries gives you the opportunity to develop increased respect for more subtle boundaries. As you shift your behavior on the basis of this learning, you reduce the amount of stress in your life and discover the benefits of honoring your personal authority.

Alice, sixty-three and a secret binge eater, had a responsible job in advertising. She felt overworked and behind in her tasks, angry, and anxious. She wondered why she wasn't given the respect she believed she deserved. One afternoon, she called me from work, and it was then that I discovered her lack of boundaries. Her door was open. Coworkers entered at will, speaking to her while she was obviously on the phone. She even accepted phone calls during our conversation.

Creating boundaries where she had none was a challenge for Alice and vital to her recovery. With fear and trepidation, she made signs for her door to let people know when she was not to be disturbed. She learned to enforce it when people came in despite the sign. She limited phone calls by politely letting people know how much time she could give them or when she would call them back. As her boundary setting became established in her workplace, she received more respect, felt less anxious, and was more effective at her job. Alice assumed going against what she thought was the office culture would bring her problems, not benefits. As she developed effective self-caring boundaries, her work experience improved. To her surprise, she also felt fewer urges to binge eat.

It's important to remember that energy surges at boundary crossings. A boundary represents someone saying no or "If you cross this boundary, everything changes."

This doesn't mean that you never cross boundaries. You cross them with permission or because you are willing to accept the consequences. An adult may be abusing her son, and the child is not your responsibility, nor do you feel you have authority to interfere, but you may do so because you can't tolerate the child's suffering. You are willing to cross that boundary knowing that the adult may well turn her anger and violence against you. You know you may need to call the police, ask for help, or take on temporary responsibility for this child.

You've crossed a boundary into a different reality than you were in a moment ago.

The ability to say no to what is not good for you is critical in honoring boundaries. This means ending your people-pleasing tendencies.

Saying no takes many forms. Your challenge in learning about boundaries includes learning how to protect your boundaries with a "no" that does the job. A shy whisper may not be enough, and an angry shout may be too much. How you say no will change depending on the occasion.

Honoring boundaries involves honesty and is unlikely to be compatible with people pleasing. If you mean, "When I finish this project," then say it. If you mean, "That activity is not something I like to do. Perhaps we could do something else another time," then say that.

People pleasing is a theme that continually comes up in eating disorder recovery. It is a major block to healthy boundary setting when you believe others cannot tolerate disappointment or adjust to your changing circumstances. You may be surprised at how friends, family, and coworkers appreciate knowing your genuine experience so they can have a more authentic relationship with you.

You have places where others are welcome, places where others must ask permission to enter, places where others are not permitted unless they are trustworthy intimates, and places that are yours alone. These can be actual physical places in your home or office, but they might also be emotions and thoughts you are not willing to share or topics of conversation you are unwilling to participate in. We all have places that are ours alone.

You may protest at this point and ask, "Where is spontaneity?" Once you are clear about boundaries, you will have more spontaneity in your life than ever before. When you know you can honor your limits, you will discover that you can give a sincere yes to what or who you want in your experience.

DAILY EXERCISES

1. Follow your breath for five minutes at least three times a day.
2. Read or recite your three affirmations twenty times each at least three times a day.
3. Write as many ways as you can think of to say no. Envision what your life would be like if you were free to say

no when and where you meant it.
4. Backtrack: Every day this week, pick a food item or a possession in your home and backtrack it. Notice how many boundaries the item or possession passed through.

CHAPTER 6
SECRETS

"How much truth can a spirit bear, how much truth can a spirit dare? . . . that became for me more and more the real measure of value."
— Friedrich Nietzsche

Carrying secrets is an enduring burden for a person with an eating disorder. You carry secrets to protect yourself from shame and yet protecting your secrets erodes your strength and self esteem and limits or damages your relationships. Releasing yourself from your secrets requires thoughtful courage and is a powerful step toward your recovery. Boundaries and secrets are inextricably entwined. When you violate boundaries and enter a forbidden zone, your sense of shame and inability to confide in a trusted person forces you to create secrets.

It's as if you thought fire was pretty and wanted to pick it like a flower. Warnings to not touch it and the heat from the flames do not register in your mind as boundary warnings. You reach to pick the flower and get burned. Your burn feels like a reproach. You feel caught, betrayed, and ashamed. You can't let anyone know of your shameful act because you fear their judgment. You want their continued admiration and respect, so you hide your burn. If anyone sees it, they might ask how you got it. You'll have to be prepared with a credible explanation.

Now you have a burdensome secret. You have to be alert to any movements that will reveal your burn, which means you can't be spontaneous and natural. Lying to your friends creates a barrier to honesty and intimacy. Your friend says, "Let's go swimming." You have to make up a lie, because in a bathing suit your burn will show. She says, "Let's take the kids to the zoo." You say yes, but insist on wearing long sleeves on a hot day. You suffer, and your companions don't understand why.

Protecting your secret reinforces your sense of shame and unworthiness. You may binge or starve to escape these feelings. The stress from protecting your secrets is ever-present.

You free yourself from your secrets by appreciating and respecting boundaries. Later we'll look at boundaries and secrets as they relate to your eating. First we need to look at how boundaries affect secrets and how secrets affect your life.

When you have a familiar feeling of anxiety, it can build into feelings of danger. To be capable of caring for yourself and having genuine confidence, you need to recognize danger signals and be ready to cope with them. The dangers you sense may be real or imagined — right now, it may be difficult for you to know the difference. Developing ways to protect yourself and get relief from your anxiety is an ongoing challenge.

Babies need love, acceptance, and reliable care to be safe and to thrive. We don't outgrow these needs, and they're satisfied throughout our lives with self-love, self acceptance, self-care, and by bringing caring and loving people into our lives.

If you had a childhood where these needs were not fulfilled, you grew up with a core of insecurity, anxiety, and fear. You may also believe you deserve to suffer because you possess some unknown but terrible flaw that sets you apart from other people. You try to keep your flaw a secret, even though you don't know exactly what it is. You try to find ways to make yourself happy and fulfilled, despite your inability to care for yourself in a healthy way. You develop an eating disorder to help you feel safe in the world. Your eating disorder is reliable and ever-present. It never says no to you. It soothes and comforts you. It's your safe haven. But you want more from life, and so you find creative (and sometimes startling and dangerous) ways to fulfill your need for love, companionship, security, and acceptance.

Laura, ashamed of her 280 pounds, keeps her size a secret. She avoids being seen by working from home. She lives in front of her computer, compulsively eating and building a virtual double life: she has a professional life that brings her income and a fantasy world where she pretends to be someone else. She has online relationships with men, sometimes using different personas to carry on several pseudo-relationships at once. Laura sounds friendly and vibrant on the phone and in her e-mails, but she avoids face-to-face meetings. She is worried that she will lose her virtual erotic relationships and long-distance love affairs as Skype video chatting grows in popularity.

Laura craves but doesn't believe she is worth admiration and acceptance. She hides what she considers to be her unworthy self and pretends to be the woman she wishes to be. Through secrets and lies, she attracts and gratifies people in her work world and her telephone and online fantasy world. She gets praise and acceptance for her professional competence. She gets intimate conversations and virtual sexual gratification from her fantasy role playing. She pleases all these people while hiding her body and genuine emotions. Because she keeps her real self a secret, she can't live openly and spontaneously or have genuine relationships. She doesn't really know what she would be like if she were free.

Stephanie, suffering from bulimia, throws herself into her life fearlessly. She seeks out risky activities like skydiving, bungee jumping, or deliberately walking alone in dark and isolated areas. She takes illegal risks by stealing and befriending people who are engaged in illegal activities. She crosses personal and legal boundaries with little or no compunction because she keeps her own vulnerability a secret from herself. She's more concerned with impressing others to shore up her insecurities about her well-being. She keeps her bingeing and purging a secret from others. Why she binges and purges is a secret she keeps from herself.

Stephanie dulls her sense of fear through her eating disorder and overwhelms her awareness with intense sensations. Danger attracts her, not because she wants to cheat death, but because she welcomes the flooding sensations as pure exhilaration and then has no room to feel other emotions. She hides her genuine experience from herself and latches on to thrills, and she feels a secret superiority about some of her antisocial or illegal activities. Yet, at the same time, keeping those activities a secret creates stress.

Madeline, alternating between bulimia and anorexia, is aware of risks she takes in rock climbing and scuba diving without adequate training and also uses recreational drugs. She relinquishes her power to make reasonable choices for herself because she puts her safety into the hands of men she believes will protect her. Because she is vulnerable to false praise and is easily seduced, she gives unreliable and sometimes exploitative men power and control in her life. She keeps her lack of qualifications a secret. She pretends she is at ease with taking drugs because she is afraid to lose the company of the man she is following. Her discomfort and insecurity are a secret. Her activities with this man are a secret from friends and family. And the reason for her eating disorder is a secret from herself.

Madeline wants protection and love. When

she over-values someone, usually a man, she feels insecure but daring and hopeful while he lures her into dangerous situations. She will also surrender to a mentor who is a moral and ethical person who wants to guide her career or personal life. Unfortunately for her, the ethical man will be concerned about being given too much power and withdraw. The unethical man has his own reasons for manipulating her. She interprets his attention as love despite her sense of worthlessness and feelings of guilt and shame that she is not competent on her own. She keeps her feelings a secret from him and her unsavory activities a secret from others.

In these examples, Laura, Stephanie, and Madeline each have a weak sense of boundaries; they can go anywhere, or they can go nowhere. What they can't do is rely on inner resiliency, because they don't know how to take responsible care of themselves in new or unpredictable situations.

Can you identify with the way these women take risks? If you can, your eating disorder seems vital to your ability to function in the world. It diffuses your awareness and authentic feelings when you can't cope with the knowledge and challenges they would bring. If any of these stories feel familiar to you then you can appreciate the anxieties Laura, Stephanie, and Madeline feel at the thought of being found out or abandoned.

If your outer life does not match your inner sense of yourself, you will continue to rely on your eating disorder to dull your anxieties and keep you focused on the pretend life you are living. Without recovery work, your eating disorder will get worse as your secrets play a larger and larger part in your daily life. When you live to please people and hide what you believe is your core unworthiness, you continually adapt and adjust your behavior to be compatible with people who have different and conflicting value systems. In order to please them all, your secrets become more complex and burdensome over time.

How do secrets relate to your life? Have you ever confided in a friend but made her swear not to tell your mother or your sister or your husband or her husband? Do you lie about who you spend time with or where you go? Do you allow your sexuality to be used socially or professionally but keep those activities secret from your family, friends, and coworkers?

When you can say yes or no based on your authentic values, the choices you make have integrity, so secrets are unnecessary. The stress of carrying secrets dissolves. You will not need an eating disorder to soothe yourself or hide feelings from yourself. You can live honestly as the woman you truly are, in all aspects of your life. If this seems unthinkable to you, you are discovering how pervasive secrets are in your life.

Your secrets can make you feel powerful and special but, if discovered, you fear they will make you an outcast or worse. Your solution to keeping your secret is bingeing or starving.

Here are some secrets you might be keeping that contribute to your need for your eating disorder.

- Stealing objects.
- Hiding embarrassing or illegal aspects of your past.
- Hiding the fact that you're taking a class or going to therapy from those closest to you because your initiative might make them angry.
- Hiding your eating disorder.

You carry secrets to protect your status quo. You believe you experience no consequences to your life or your relationships if no one finds out your secrets. It's similar to throwing up after a binge or running hard and long to burn off calories. It's like adding fat to your body from overeating and getting regular liposuction treatments. You believe keeping your secrets will protect you from unwanted consequences.

Trying to avoid consequences brings unintended consequences. For example, you are certain that revealing your secrets would disrupt your life, bring you and others pain, and cause others to shun you. But by keeping secrets you hide a portion of your life. Friends, family, coworkers, and classmates have no idea that the person they believe is you is actually a stranger in disguise. You feel lonely and insecure because the woman they are relating to isn't you, and they may feel betrayed when they find out you've been untruthful.

Your secrets create barriers. They haunt you because you must be alert to not let your secret slip through word or action or appearance. If a hint of your secret comes through, you must be quick to find a lie to cover it up. Living with the possibility of someone discovering your secrets at any time causes you to rely more on your eating disorder to overwhelm your growing anxieties.

When you disregard a boundary to gratify

your yearnings for a better, safer, more interesting or satisfying way of living, you change a balance in your life and relationships. If you believe the people in your life cannot tolerate and adjust to your changes, you may make your move in secret. You don't realize that creating another secret perpetuates your suffering and your eating disorder.

Recovery includes freeing yourself from the pattern of creating secrets. The pathway to this freedom requires your willingness to look through your rationalizations, false beliefs, and eating-disordered thinking, and see how you actually live. Once you see your own patterns, you can dare to make changes.

A classic fairy tale goes like this: The miller's daughter, an ordinary girl, must spin straw into gold or the king will kill her. If she succeeds, however, he will make her his queen. It took me many years of living to understand that he was not a cruel and selfish man or she a hapless victim.

We all are called upon in this life to spin our straw into gold. We accumulate baggage (illnesses, sorrows, consequences of mistaken judgment, and more). Keeping this baggage a secret becomes a burden that can destroy our chance for a rich life. We need to spin it into gold. We need to learn from it and grow beyond it, so we are empowered to live a life of quality.

You have secrets that a few people don't know about. You have secrets that you think no one knows about. You have secrets that, indeed, no one does know about. And you have secrets that even you don't know about, secrets from yourself.

Here are clues that indicate you have secrets from yourself. You have blanks in your childhood memories and don't know the difference between stories you were told and what you actually experienced. You hide that you go blank for moments in conversation. You go blank or get distracted during a movie or while reading and are certain you can fill in what you missed and follow the story line.

Seemingly insignificant things, like an object out of place or someone spilling something, arouses fear or anger inside you. You feel the urge to leave social or professional gatherings, or you actually do leave, because you are too nervous to stay. Yet, you can't say specifically what's wrong. What's happening is that your present day experience triggers a feeling that comes from a past experience, a feeling you are incapable of dealing with. The feeling you had in your original experience comes roaring up, but the actual experience remains a mystery.

Christina, a single professional in her forties, lived in an unkempt home when she was actively bulimic. Her mess was her secret, and she did not allow visitors. During one phase of her recovery, however, she poured hours of daily energy into cleaning and organizing her living space. She went from not caring at all about her home to becoming meticulous. She still could not have visitors.

Christina's secret from herself was that she was afraid if she let something get out of place, it would unleash uncontrollable forces in the world, including her bulimia. Below that secret was another. As good as her life was, she was afraid that she could lose it and bring back her chaotic childhood where she was loved but ignored and unappreciated. That fear was part of the underlying secret that fueled her eating disorder.

Christina discovered through recovery that she had developed competence and sturdiness. She learned she had the personal power to prevent a fall back into the painful and inescapable ways of her childhood. Christina replaced her bulimia with her own competence and faith in herself.

Underlying secrets may be well hidden from you but not from the people around you. Are your sexual experiences vague or difficult to remember? Are you aware when you are having sex but remember little or nothing afterwards? Clara, a twenty-one-year-old bride, kept her bulimia, compulsive eating, and occasional bouts with anorexia a secret. She was shocked and amazed that her new husband remembered their sexual activities and wanted to talk about them. She had no idea it was possible to remember such things and was horrified that he did. His wanting to talk about their sexual activities broke a psychic law for her. Her secret from herself was so powerful she didn't know it existed.

When you have secrets that you know about, you also have secrets that you don't know about. When you live a life full of secrets, they seem normal to you, including the emotional burden of keeping them from yourself.

It's not unusual for someone with an eating disorder to have surprising and inexplicable physical sensations, like trembling, chills, nausea, dizziness, lightheadedness, or sudden sweating — all with no medical basis. Your eating disorder blocks the connection between your feelings and physical sensations. You don't understand your physical symptoms and will go to food to ease your physical sensations, even nausea.

Washi, forty-eight and divorced, lived alone in Los Angeles during her first three months of recovery from bulimia. One night, she was awakened by a big thump on her bed. She noticed her bed was shaking. Her first thought was: earthquake! She looked at her hanging mobile, and it was still. Washi was confused as her bed continued to shake. Then she realized her body was shaking. She lay quietly, watching her body shake, and she thought to herself, "I suppose if I were feeling this, I'd be terrified." This was a breakthrough for Washi, because she saw herself using her body to avoid her emotions.

Trudy, fifty-five, eats compulsively. She's married with three grown sons and is quick to apologize when her husband or friends hurt or offend her. She doesn't understand why her sons are angry with her for not sticking up for herself. Trudy says she knows she makes mistakes, and if someone criticizes or insults her, she is probably in the wrong. She does what she can to make the other person feel better. Trudy often offers her family and guests food and will binge alone in the kitchen while she prepares it.

Both Washi and Trudy share a lack of knowledge about themselves. Washi is discovering that her thinking mind, her feelings, and her body sensations are at times severely disconnected. Trudy has yet to discover that she is unconsciously blocking her feelings. Their true nature and authentic responses are secrets from themselves.

Because you avoid knowing your secrets through lies and oblivion doesn't mean other people don't notice when you respond oddly. They may even count on your disconnection from yourself to exploit you. Trudy's husband takes advantage of her people-pleasing ways to get special treatment for himself and his friends. Her sons notice her inappropriate people-pleasing responses and alternate between worrying about her well-being and being frustrated with her. Trudy's current methods of caring for herself do not protect her from exploitation. And they prevent her from self-knowledge and hope for changing her status quo. Her eating disorder just perpetuates this unhappy situation.

If any of these stories or descriptions trigger images and associations from your own life, you may have secrets from yourself. If you feel anxiety or anger or a desire to stop reading, something in this section is touching a sensitive area in you that wants to remain protected and hidden. If you have an urge to move into your eating disorder after reading this, you can be sure you are trying to keep some information out of your awareness.

Once you unburden yourself of secrets, you can align yourself more fully with your recovery. You develop the necessary strength and resources you need to deal well with your life.

This does not mean that you're going to blurt out your secrets indiscriminately. Secrets often have to do with shame, and bringing genuine understanding and forgiveness to your situation by working through them with a trusted person can dissolve your burden. You don't have to relieve yourself of your painful secret by placing a new burden on someone else. You can relieve yourself of a secret without going public with it. Keep in mind there's a difference between what is secret and what is private.

Here are a few questions that will help you examine your pattern of guarding secrets. Answer the questions now, and review your answers in a few weeks or months. They will help you understand how your secrets influence your life and also show you that you've been more courageous in your recovery than you know.

1. What topics can you not talk about?
2. What people must you avoid?
3. What questions must you not ask?
4. What lifestyle seems good to you but impossible to ever have?
5. What activities can you not do or join?
6. In what situations must you be silent and defer to others?
7. What fulfilling ways of living can other people have but not you?
8. What rules prevent you from making your life better?
9. What do your family and friends expect and assume about you that are not compatible with your sense of yourself?
10. What are your hopes and interests that would surprise people?

Without your conscious awareness, you may accept people into your life who will expect and enforce your unsatisfying way of living. They can become your abusers or controlling influences because, in a world where you have secrets from yourself, you acquiesce to what they expect and demand of you. You can't imagine saying no and letting yourself and them learn what might emerge from you if you were free.

Recovery work involves challenging your own belief system so you can move forward with your life. Your new assertiveness may disappoint or shock others. You may be frightened because you don't know yourself what to expect. Whatever their response, you need to be capable of dealing with it. Before your authentic self can emerge from under the load of secrets and routines, you need time and space to breathe and make room for that emergence.

Some people in your life may not be able to accept your changing, and a parting of ways will be necessary. You may also discover that some people you thought were controlling you with their expectations and assumptions lay down their own burdens as you take on more responsibilities. You won't know who is disgruntled or dismissive of your emergent self or who is delighted, relieved, or encouraging until you move toward your own authenticity.

Your husband may want you to be his submissive wife who follows the pattern you both have established over the years. He may not be able to accept your changes and the marriage flounders or ends. But your husband may be thrilled and delighted by your growth that results in new opportunities and challenges for you both. A dull marriage bogged down by routine can become vibrant and alive as you take on new activities and share new adventures. Basically, you don't know what will happen to your relationship and neither does he until you move toward your own authenticity. You know that by making these changes you are freeing yourself of secrets and your need for your eating disorder. You are saving your own life.

If you are still reading this, you may be ready to tamper with your unconscious system of guarding secrets. Shame, guilt, and fear stop you from recognizing your ability to discover your strength, resiliency, stamina, courage, and determination. If you recognized these qualities in yourself and had access to them, you could expose your secrets and challenge the system that limits your life. Your eating disorder is part of that system.

Your recovery rests in finding those positive elements in your psyche and developing the courage and skills to use them. When you use your eating disorder to block your anxiety, you're also blocking the glimmering awareness of your strengths.

143

As you examine your secrets, you build your awareness and ability to tolerate the reality of your situation. This frees your creativity so you can discover or develop new and better ways to cope with stress and anxiety. Crossing boundaries that create the burden of secrets will be less inviting. You will recognize both the boundary and the cost of crossing it. You will trust and honor yourself more as you carry with you less that is based on fantasy and more that is based on what will truly benefit you. You'll start making wise decisions that change your life for the better.

This work on boundaries and secrets is critical. I hope you continue to return to these chapters as a part of your normal way of living. The words on the pages will not change, but you will have been healing, and you will experience the words and the exercises differently.

EXERCISE

1. Expand your breathing exercises to ten minutes.
2. Read or recite your three affirmations twenty times each at least three times a day.
3. Write about a challenge in your life.

In your mind, ask for direction or guidance from someone who is meaningful to you. This can be anyone — someone you know, a celebrity, a historical figure, or a fictional character. Relax, and allow yourself to be surprised by the answers that flow through your pen. You will be opening resources in yourself that may have been shut down for a long time.

4. Backtrack a secret. Follow the trail of your secret back in time, noticing how it influences your actions and your relationships. Go back to when you acquired the secret, and then before that. Find clues that show you why you harbored the secret and why you continue to carry it with you today.

CHAPTER 7
CHALLENGES TO EATING WELL

"The only devils in this world are those running around inside our own hearts, and that is where all our battles should be fought."

— Gandhi

Now that you have a better understanding of boundaries and have gained strength in tolerating personal discoveries, you can venture into the highly sensitive subject of food and how you eat. I invite you to look carefully at what function eating serves in your life beyond physical nourishment. You are looking to build an approach to food that lessens fear and urgency, and creates more peace and pleasure.

With awareness you enlist cooperation from your mind and body simultaneously so you develop an integrated internal support system for changing your eating style. You can rely on your increased ability to be

146

present and the resiliency you've developed by following the exercises in this book. You can rely on these qualities as you explore healthier ways of eating and not eating, with accompanying exercises that emphasize kindness and reassurance.

When you have your own internal support system, you listen to your emotional cravings and body yearnings with understanding and have the ability to make wise choices. You say no to what is not good for you and yes to what nourishes you. You are able to discern and respect the differences between what your heart needs and what your body needs.

Your eating patterns define the name of your eating disorder, but you don't need a diagnosis to know that your way of eating stops you from living a more full life. You may qualify for a specific or nonspecific eating disorder diagnosis. But you are not your eating disorder. You are not a diagnosis. *Your eating patterns do not define you as a person.* You are a woman suffering from an eating disorder. The eating disorder can go away but you will remain.

Our culture and language usage defines men and women (sadly, now children too) as fat. The correct recognition of fat is that it's a substance within your body. For example, you say, "I have an allergy." You don't say, "I *am* an allergy." You say, "I have a sore throat." You don't say, "I am a sore throat." And you can say, "I carry fat." You don't have to say, "I am fat." Fat is a substance, not an identity.

You may believe that your relationship with food does define you. Do you suffer from an eating disorder or are you an eating disorder? Do you say, "I am an anorexic," or do you say, "I suffer from anorexia"?

These are important distinctions because what you say your ears hear and your mind remembers. If you define yourself by your illness, you erode your real identity. Your definition of yourself as an eating disorder can mire you in negative self-perceptions, harsh judgments, and feelings of futility and despair.

I invite you to suspend your beliefs about your eating and your negative self-definition. You do this the same way you suspend your beliefs about reality when you watch a film or read a novel. Let yourself suspend your belief in your current time and surroundings. Accept, on a temporary basis, the possibility of being in a different time and place. You are in London in the year 1853, and you're walking the streets with Sherlock Holmes and Watson on the trail of

Moriarty. Or maybe you are in the far future on the starship Enterprise, hurtling through space at a speed faster than light to save planet Earth from invaders. You have the ability to suspend your belief. Do this with your own definition of you.

In this open-minded place, look at the way you eat and how you might gradually make adjustments in your psychological and emotional attachments to food.

When you feel inevitable tightening and reluctance to do this exploration, do this "Be Present for Another Minute" exercise — I call it PAM for short. Watch your breath as you shake your shoulders, do three neck rolls, shake your legs, and flex your feet. You will discover that when you want to shut this book or run away, doing a three- to five-minute PAM will help you stay present and bear your feelings.

Pay attention to how you feel right now. Having read the first few paragraphs of this chapter, are you excited, scared, hopeful, looking for fast answers, or looking for another diet regime with familiar grim determination? Whatever you are feeling, you still have this book open. Great. Give yourself credit for this, and stay with your experience.

If you feel too anxious or angry or excited

to continue this chapter, pause and breathe. Do a PAM. Be aware of your body and your physical presence. Your whole person is made up of your mind, feelings, body, and spirit. Be still and become aware of your whole self. Read the following two sentences three times a day along with your breathing, shoulder shake, and neck roll exercise.

1. My body needs fuel and nourishment to survive and function.
2. I eat adequate and appropriate amounts of food daily that contain necessary nourishment for my body.

Watch your body. Pay attention to how your body feels.

Keep reading, and whenever your feelings get strong, rather than pressing forward despite your feelings or stopping to avoid your feelings, pause and do PAM. Then come back to the words you know you need to hear.

If a person eats too much or not enough food, or the food lacks adequate nourishment or contains toxins, something is amiss. What benefits do you get from eating in a way that does not support living a long and healthy life? What good comes to you by denying yourself healthful food at appropriate times and in appropriate amounts on a regular basis?

Keep breathing and doing shoulder rolls as we proceed. Try to keep your emotions even enough so you can continue reading and thinking. When we get to the actual food conversations, you will be sensitive, vulnerable, and accustomed to your own self-criticisms and anxieties. So hang in there and know that I know you are being brave by reading this chapter now.

You retreat into your self-criticism when you hear "It's the diet that fails and not you." You are certain this is a lie designed to make you feel better about yourself, and hearing it makes you feel worse. Keep breathing and keep doing your body shakes and shoulder rolls because the diet failure statement is true. But if you believe this statement you feel left with nothing at all. If you are failing, then you can try again with another diet. But if diets fail, you have no choice except to be miserable forever. Something is missing in this logic. This kind of thinking leaves out the nature of an eating disorder and why you are in its tenacious grip. There's a protective force at work within you that you don't understand, but which is real and creates your rigid or chaotic, controlled or out-of-control way of eating.

You reach a psychological and emotional place where this force seems to compel you to eat or not to eat, sabotaging your health, appearance, energy, relationships, and life goals. You feel helpless to resist the urges and often don't even try. Most of the time you may be eager to indulge your eating disorder behaviors, only to feel unhappy and disappointed after the fact.

Look at your symptoms and what they might mean. You know from your own experience and from your discoveries in the previous chapters that eating disorder behavior is not about hunger. Often a person with an eating disorder doesn't recognize the sensation of hunger. If hunger isn't your cue to eat and satiation your cue to stop, what are your cues?

Here's an example of what might be happening: a slight nervous sensation just below your shoulders in your upper arms; a leaden feeling in your abdomen; a prickling behind your forehead and a slight throbbing behind your ears; a quivering in your upper thighs. All these sensations can send you to food. These and other mild feelings are like low, tiny tremblers alerting you to an earthquake that is coming. You eat to prevent the earthquake.

The sensations can be so slight you may not recognize them. You just know you need to eat. An important part of your recovery work is to recognize these sensations and stay with them for longer periods of time before resorting to your eating disorder behavior. As you develop a tolerance for these sensations and an understanding of what they mean, you discover they pass like a wave.

You may eat until you are numb and immobile or until you reach a physical and emotional state you can tolerate. Then you may nibble or graze throughout the day to maintain that state. Perhaps you can't eat enough to reach a safe emotional place. Then you may eat until you can't hold any more food. You throw up so you can continue eating. You have some relief while you are actually eating, but you must keep eating far more than your body will allow.

You may go the other way and avoid your feelings by going into starvation mode. You strive to reach the ethereal high that comes with a starving brain. You need to remain empty and get smaller so your body cannot experience unbearable sensations. At times, the biological imperative to stay alive will push you into an uncontrollable devouring binge. You eat voraciously, throwing up as often as you can. You stop from exhaustion or because you pass out.

Your emotional eating may not be as dramatic as these examples. You may go about your normal routine, using food as an automatic cruise control on your feelings. You eat what you need as often as you need to maintain a tolerable emotional state. You might munch on cookies or nuts or eat cheese and crackers to get you through a work assignment or a conversation.

These eating episodes are not based on hunger. They are based on your trying to take care of yourself in the only way you know how. You don't know why you need to eat this way. You do know that you can't resist. You may believe your reason is that you are bizarre, bad, disgusting, horrible, unlovable, crazy, or a "thing" that needs to be hidden from other people.

Someone who doesn't have an eating disorder might still comfort themselves with food during a time of stress. The difference between that person and you is that you don't have other means of comforting yourself. Your extremes in eating are routine. Without your comfort food, you feel more desperate, angry, or frightened than you can bear.

Please, right now, pay attention to your breath and then say to yourself, "My ways of using food do not define my identity or my character. They are symptoms of my eating disorder. They are my attempt to take care of myself."

Once you understand this, you see why diet programs don't work. Taking away or limiting your access to what takes care of you will leave you too vulnerable and anxious. Diets don't take this into consideration. Neither do exercise programs or weight loss surgeries. These interventions make sense only when you consider food consumption and weight gain, not when you consider the emotional need for an eating disorder. When your ways of eating change and you lose weight, you are emotionally unprotected. If you have no solid backup system in place, no awareness, no presence, and no skills to care for yourself, you will go back to your old proven methods. You call it a relapse, gain or lose weight, and feel like a failure.

You didn't fail. The program failed because it didn't take into consideration what your weight and ways of eating do for your psychological sense of well-being. The diet program didn't address the fact that you would be emotionally helpless without your old ways of functioning. If you want to change your eating style and body size, you need to build a sturdy internal psychological structure that allows you to respond in a healthy and self-caring way to your emotional challenges. Without that in place you will, quite naturally, reach for what you know will work — your eating disorder.

This book is designed to help you build what you need to live well. It's not about diet and exercise, although a good diet and exercise are parts of any healthy lifestyle.

This book is about your becoming sturdy of mind, heart, and soul so that you don't need the eating disorder. As you incorporate the exercises into your daily life, you learn what underlies the physical and emotional sensations that send you to your eating disorder behaviors. At the same time, you develop inner resources that allow you to respond differently to your stress. Food becomes a source of nourishment and, at times, a source of entertainment and celebration. But it is no longer the rescuer in your life.

EATING PLAN #1

A basic healthy approach to food begins with a substantial high quality and nourishing breakfast that includes all food groups. You can tweak the contents of this breakfast over time, but your main criteria are that it be substantial and healthful. This sets up your body to "break its fast" from the night before. Your metabolism wakes up. Your body now knows that you have fed it. It's not going to be pushed into starvation mode, which can switch your feelings into cravings and your actions into binges.

This approach includes a lunch consisting of all food groups. It may be of moderate or substantial size, depending on your level of physical activity. The days where I play on the beach or go for a long walk are days when I have a substantial lunch. Days where I sit writing I have a moderate lunch.

Since you are probably not accustomed to eating a substantial breakfast, your body may still feel satisfied midday. You don't have hunger signals, but on this plan you eat lunch anyway. You eat moderate servings of healthful, fresh, clean, nontoxic food.

You may have to press against old thinking, like, "Why waste calories and eat when I am not hungry? Why not wait and save the room and the calories so I can binge later with fewer consequences?" "Why should I eat if I don't want to? I can lose more weight if I don't eat." That kind of thinking reinforces the starvation cycle where your body does not trust that it will be fed adequately again. The emptiness builds until you click into binge mode to make up for the past starvation experience and the certainty that another famine will come soon.

You eat a light dinner that includes all food groups. Giving your body adequate nourishment in a timely manner changes the body's experience. You break the starvation cycle. Eventually, your body trusts that it will be fed.

This plan includes two healthful snacks a day, preferably about two hours before lunch and dinner. Don't go more than four hours without eating (hungry or not). Don't use artificial sweeteners of any kind or in any form. Once you befriend your body and earn your own trust, your food choices become more appropriate for the weight that is right for your frame.

If this discussion is bringing up anxiety or anger or hopeless feelings, please take a PAM break and come back to this chapter. Sometimes even talking about a change in your way of eating can trigger your eating disorder. If your feelings are strong, do the exercises and activities that have been most helpful to you. Then pace yourself based on your willingness and stamina. Nothing in this book needs to be done immediately — except one thing: begin your recovery.

As you move into this food plan, there will be times when you want to binge or restrict to cover feelings you can't bear. You can't binge well because you are adequately nourished. You can't restrict well because your body likes being nourished. You will be tempted to force yourself back to your old ways by discounting what your body wants and needs. This is a time to be kind to yourself and practice your breathing.

There's no way around your main challenge. You have to bear your feelings. Recognizing a sense of hunger, appreciating a meal, and eating a balanced meal alone or with others are major achievements for a person with an eating disorder. Your work is to develop the strength to gradually bear what you can without relying on the eating disorder.

EXPLORING YOUR EATING DISORDER URGES:
A GRADUAL APPROACH TO AWARENESS AND STRENGTH

Pause Exercise Before You Act on an Eating Disorder Urge

Week 1: Pause. Pay attention to how you feel in the midst of an urge. Find out what the intolerable feels like, if just for a moment. Stop yourself for half a minute before you act out. The pause will give you a glimpse of the emotional state you want to avoid. A glimpse is all you need now.

Week 2: Continue to pause, but this week, add your breathing exercise. Pay attention to where your breath moves through your body during your urge. Observe your body in detail. Become acquainted with your physical sensations.

Week 3: Continue as you did in week 2, and add an activity. Write, draw, sing, dance, or walk during the time you postpone acting on your eating disorder urge.

This timeframe is arbitrary. Find a schedule that is gradual for you. You might add the next level in two weeks rather than one. You might need to go back to the first and begin again. All these possibilities are fine. You are working toward extending time between your eating disorder urges and your eating disorder behaviors.

You experience great passion in acting out your eating disorder. The feelings you experience during the pause will also be passionate and strong. You may cry or rage or be afraid. You may remember past hurts, losses, or unfilled yearnings. You may feel you are locked in a permanent state of profound loneliness where no one could ever find you. You may tremble with craving.

You eat or starve to avoid these feelings. As you develop your tolerance of them without food-related behavior, you can be more sensitive to what your body experiences. You can bring more compassion to yourself during intense emotional states. Once you begin to experience the feelings beneath the urges, you have made great strides in your recovery.

At this point, you appreciate that food is only for your body, and you have to find other ways to cope with your powerful emotions. You are close to knowing how hunger feels.

Carol, thirty-seven years old and suffering from binge eating since she was eleven, called me one afternoon with a delight in her voice I had never heard before. She said, "I found out what hunger is!" She explained that she felt a strange feeling in her abdomen, like a tickle. It didn't hurt, but it didn't go away. She was in a stage in her recovery where she didn't go more than four hours without eating. She used time cues for meals and snacks because she didn't know what hunger was.

On this day, however, she felt that tickle. She saw that it was about ten minutes beyond four hours, so she made herself a cold chicken plate with a small salad. She said, "I loved it. My body loved it. I was hungry. I ate, and then I wasn't hungry anymore!"

If you have an eating disorder, it's likely that you don't know what hunger is. You may know the feeling of starvation and famine, but not normal hunger. Regardless of the nature of your eating disorder, you are not consuming or avoiding food because of hunger issues.

Martha, thirty-three and in the medical profession, eats compulsively. She says, "But

I'm hungry all the time. I love food." She doesn't understand she wants food constantly for emotional stability, not to satisfy physical hunger.

A woman with an eating disorder, whether she suffers from anorexia, bulimia, or compulsive overeating, finds sitting at a table for a meal with others stressful.

Shalini compulsively overeats and has binge eating episodes almost every night. She doesn't want to waste calories by eating with her family or friends at a restaurant. She wants to save those calories for her private eating. She worries that a binge eating episode will sneak up on her. She is afraid she won't be able to fake eating normally in public.

Keira suffers from anorexia. She wears layers of clothes to give the impression she is bigger than she is. She wears flowing long sleeves to hide her bony arms. She tells her dinner companions she ate a large snack earlier to justify her tiny food order. Keira cuts her food into tiny pieces and moves the pieces around her plate to give the impression that she is eating. She puts food in her mouth, pretends to chew, and spits the food into her napkin. She has many ploys to reduce her tension and get away from the pressure to eat. She spills her plate and refuses a replacement. The drama helps her push away food, distracts her from her hunger, and breaks the tension she feels based on real or imagined judgments directed toward her. She may find fault with the meal so she can send it back to the kitchen. She may pick a fight with someone at the table, and cry as if she were wounded to justify leaving the table or the restaurant. Keira's tears are real. She is in torment.

Claire suffers from bulimia. Her first concern about eating at a restaurant with her family is the layout of the bathrooms. She goes to the ladies' room immediately to discover if it's one room with a door she can lock or if it's cubicles. If it's a one-room bathroom, she relaxes. If it's cubicles, she will have to plan her eating carefully so she can allow time to throw up and wait for everyone to leave so no one can identify her when she emerges. She orders foods she can throw up easily and quietly. During dinner Claire will leave the table several times to purge.

If the stress to appear normal becomes too great, Shalini, Keira, or Claire will find an excuse to leave. They will fake an illness, lie about forgotten appointments, or create an argument so they can storm out. These three women are crippled by an internal war of control between a malnourished mind that distorts reality and healthy body urgings that strive for survival.

Their internal pressure to behave as if they were normal eaters plays havoc with their emotions. Shalina feels shame because she's certain her brother saw her eat noodles too fast and spill sauce on her blouse. Keira feels frightened and angry because she believes her family brought her to the restaurant to control her and force her to eat and get fat. Claire is worried that she's harmed relationships by leaving the table so often. She's also determined never to return to that restaurant because the bathroom didn't accommodate her purging needs.

All these women may feel lightheaded or have cramps. They want to be alone to recover their equilibrium, either by eating more and purging or by pushing themselves hard on a treadmill.

At this stage in their eating disorders, they are far from eating with an appreciation for taste and nourishment. They see food as a substance to control, or it will control them. Their ability to befriend and nourish themselves develops in recovery, but not all at once.

Healthy, peaceful, happy eating is a goal. Eating for hunger and pleasant satisfaction is based on different motivations from eating based on eating disorder urges. In health, you eat with a sense of pleasure. You give yourself needed nourishment. Your body enjoys taking in the food. Your belly calmly welcomes and receives a meal with no cramping, tension, or bloating. You savor flavors as you chew and swallow at a moderate speed. At the same time, you are able to speak and listen to others. You are flexible and open with your attention. You hear what others are saying, respond to them while enjoying your meal, and delight in sharing the experience.

If you are alone, you appreciate your surroundings while you are eating. You think, feel, and are present for your experience. You are not obsessed with the food. You are not flooded with eating sensations. You are not mindless while you are eating. You remain present.

Yes, sometimes you grab a snack on the run. Yes, sometimes you eat at your desk while going over paperwork. Yes, you find yourself in a situation where you feel required to eat, for social or family reasons, a meal that is not among your favorites. These are not ideal situations, but they happen in life. And when they do, you are able to maintain your emotional equilibrium.

If you have an eating disorder, here's a series of activities you can use to prepare for unexpected food challenges or surprising events that trigger your eating disorder behaviors. They strengthen your ability to tolerate disruptions in what you expect to be normal routines. They help you develop resiliency so you can adapt to changing conditions. I borrow the word "jibe" to describe them. Jibe is a word taken from sailing. It's when the boom shifts fast and hard from one side of the boat to the other forcing the boat to suddenly change direction.

1. Learn to jibe by using your non-dominant hand to:
   • brush your teeth
   • hold the sponge when you are washing dishes
   • use your computer mouse
   • unlock your door with your key
   • write or draw
2. When you are ready to jibe while eating, hold your fork or spoon with your non-dominant hand.

Use your imagination to find more ways you can "jibe." Get off the bus one stop before your regular stop, and walk the rest of the way. Park a block or more away from your destination and walk. Take a different route to a routine destination. Sleep on the other side of the bed. Switch storage drawers in your kitchen, bedroom, office, or garage.

These exercises will startle your mind, emotions, and body in a simple and non-threatening way that doesn't relate to food at all. Jibing in your ordinary life forces you to focus and practice being present. By upsetting routine daily habits, you enliven parts of your brain that have been asleep. You open your imagination to new possibilities that can surprise you. You feel more alert and alive. You nurture your sense of humor and laugh more. You become comfortable with being awkward and clumsy when trying something new. You have a "game" you can share with other people. You remember, or learn for the first time, how to play. Your body, mind, and spirit become more flexible and more confident in new situations. The jibing exercises help you prepare for changes that you will make in your eating patterns when that time arrives. It may help you make gradual changes now.

A mindful eating practice helps you be present and mindful not only with food, but in many other areas of your life. The following exercise uses the intricacies of a raisin to show you the range of sensory and emotional experience you can have with food, unrelated to eating disorder compulsions.

Give yourself fifteen minutes with one raisin. Look at it carefully from all angles. Pay attention to the sensation in your eyes. Hold it gently in your hand. Feel every distinct aspect of it. Pay attention to the sensations in your fingers and hand. Lift it to your nose and smell it thoroughly. Pay attention to the sensations in your nostrils. Put it in your mouth. Do not chew. Roll it around the inside of your mouth. Explore it with your tongue. Pay attention to the sensations in your mouth. Bite down once. Feel the juiciness and experience the flavor. Pay attention to how you experience taste and wetness.

Bring mindful eating into your life by giving yourself a "mindful bite" at any meal. This can stop a binge. With this exercise, you remind yourself that food has taste, texture, and distinctive qualities to explore and appreciate.

Another way to expand your appreciation of food is to have a quiet meal. Once a week, give yourself a pleasant and balanced meal in silence — no music, phone, TV, computer, reading, or company.

Lay out your meal as you would for a respected guest. Sit at the table and eat.

Put down your utensil after each mouthful. Chew thoroughly and swallow. Only pick up your fork or spoon when you feel that your last mouthful has reached your stomach. Continue until you believe you have reached the point when your body has had "enough."

Eating your way through a quiet meal can bring up strong feelings. Write them down immediately after the meal. By doing this, you strengthen your ability to tolerate a difficult feeling, even discover a feeling. The more you can tolerate your own experience, the less you will need the numbing or soothing of your eating disorder.

This practice helps you learn what you ask of food. If you follow these instructions, you will eat for body hunger only. Your emotions will be unaddressed. You receive important insight when you discover how many feelings remain raw or aching after your body has received enough food for its needs. Recognizing these feelings and what you've been asking food to do for you emotionally can be a difficult experience, but it will help you make great strides in your eating disorder recovery.

To increase your mindful awareness of food, do the backtracking exercise with a trigger or binge food. The exercise will help break your sense of isolation as you realize the myriad connections you have with people you will never know. These are the farmers who grew the food and others, who trucked it, packaged it, processed it, and sold it to you.

You are learning that when you feel an irresistible urge or craving for a food or for an eating disorder behavior, the food or behavior is not your real desire. Pause and ask yourself what you want. This backtracking exercise on binge food helps you see through your craving to what you genuinely want and helps you get it.

For example, if you are craving sweets, bring more "sweetness" into your life. Experiment with your options. You could hold a stuffed animal or get a hand massage. You could volunteer to walk dogs at a rescue shelter to experience unconditional affection and appreciation.

Another option is to take a tip from France in the 1880s and get yourself a poupée de poche (a doll for your pocket). This could be a small, sweet doll or something similar that comforts you. You can put your hand in your pocket at any time to feel that reassuring presence.

If you crave something crunchy, you want to bite down hard on something like chips and hear the sound as well as feel the sensation. You want to make an impact and know it. So bring more physicality into your life. Learn woodcraft where you use a hammer, nails, a screwdriver, and a drill to make noise and repair things. Garden in your own yard, help a neighbor, or volunteer in a community garden. Dig into the soil. Cut and prune plants. Feel a shovel in your hands as it bites into the ground.

Do you want to bite down into a deeper way of experiencing your career or your environment or your relationships? Experiment with going deeper. Learn about the structure of your home or the history of your local community. Find out about details in your neighborhood you take for granted. What kinds of trees and plants do you see every day? Learn about them. What kinds of birds or insects are part of your environment? Learn about them, too. And when you are ready, learn about the people in your immediate vicinity. What are their names? What's important to them? What makes them smile? Find ways to go deeper.

If you feel yourself asking, "How can I do

all this? Who has the time?" instead ask how much time your eating disorder requires of you. In doing these exercises on a regular basis, you are moving your energy away from your eating disorder activities and into your recovery activities.

Be mindful about your physical needs and take the initiative to create the right conditions for your own healthy eating. Stock nutritious foods in your home — fresh fruits and vegetables, wholesome proteins, beans, whole grains, flavorful herbs, and healthful oils, like olive oil and grapeseed oil. Keep your mindful eating a priority. Create an environment that offers you quality food to enjoy in a mindful eating way. You may feel frustrated when you crave your binge foods, but at the same time, your mindful choices comfort you and hold you through the passing of your emotional wave. You experience relief and delight when you crave a sweet binge, struggle to resist, and discover that you can eat a banana in a mindful way as the craving fades.

You may find yourself frightened because you've waited too long to eat and now your hunger is pushing you toward a binge. But then you remember you placed a set meal in your refrigerator or freezer that is just right for this occasion. With relief and a sense of pride that you created this quality option, you give yourself a pleasant and adequate meal.

You don't have to become a health food purist, but in the beginning, your maltreated body is like an animal in a rescue shelter. It has been taken out of an environment of neglect, deprivation, and abuse and is in a temporary holding place; not sure of what is going to happen, being more familiar with bad than good. Your body needs a lot of TLC before it's healthy and strong and knows it can trust you to feed it well and regularly.

Once you earn your own trust, you can relax with confidence because you know you are, at last, in a good, caring, loving, and responsible "home." You'll fear less and smile more. You won't have to binge to ward off your physical certainty of imminent starvation because you trust that you will be fed nourishing food on a regular basis. You won't have to starve to be tiny, invisible, and safe. You're okay.

Again you are faced with boundaries and limits. Serve yourself adequate portions of foods — not too much or too little, but the right amount for your body, your needs of the moment, and your true hunger level.

Measure out your food, especially if you

are going to eat on the run or while you are working or multitasking in any way. Your task can distract you from the amount of food you are eating. You can forget to eat or eat too much.

You don't need to always weigh and measure your food to keep portions appropriate. Invest in some pretty or fun dishes that are the right size for your food. Salad plates may be more appropriate for dinners. Tiny salt dishes might be more appropriate for high calorie snacks, like nuts. Small rice bowls might be more appropriate for cereal. This also teaches your eyes to recognize appropriate portions.

When eating out, you can use this portion recognition to give yourself reasonable servings on your plate and put the remainder in a take-out carton or an empty plate on the table for others to share if they wish. Order half portions or split a main course with another person.

You don't have to be afraid of buffet tables. At a buffet, walk through the entire display of offerings without a plate in your hands to see what choices you will make in advance. Plan the amounts you need to make a reasonable plate for yourself. When you have your plan, go through the line. You've bypassed the urges that surge with each surprise you find in the buffet. You had your surprise without a plate. Now you are free to choose what is right for you.

You are learning, as you come out of the eating disorder haze, that eating or not eating is only part of your life. With more healing, strength, and hope, your life blossoms.

DAILY EXERCISES

1. Follow your breath for five minutes at least three times a day.
2. Read or recite three affirmations twenty times each at least three times a day. See Appendix A, "Affirmations."
3. Write about making food portion decisions. Write about giving yourself "sweet" and "crunchy, bite down" experiences unrelated to food.
4. Backtrack what you are wearing today. Every day, take some time to look at the clothing and accessories on your body. Trace one or more items back to how you acquired them and what that experience meant to you at the time. This will give you an appreciation for the associations you are carrying with you and how you made decisions in the past that affect

you today. Find more activities related
to boundaries in Appendix B.

CHAPTER 8
CONTEMPLATIONS ON
EATING A MEAL

" 'Well,' said Pooh, 'what I like best,' and then he had to stop and think. Because although Eating Honey was a very good thing to do, there was a moment just before you began to eat it which was better than when you were, but he didn't know what it was called."
— A. A. Milne, The House on Pooh Corner

Bingeing, starving, grazing, purging, and stuffing food can be such familiar routines to you that they become mindless rituals.

Marcia, a thirty-three-year-old graduate student, skips meals and instead snacks while she studies. She eats through bags of chips while studying and is surprised when she closes her book and finds herself surrounded by empty plastic bags and chip crumbs. Her chip eating while studying is her mindless ritual. However, Marcia learned to use mindful ceremonies to develop more calm and healthful ways of eating.

Mindful practices that honor health and life are rooted in many cultures and religions throughout the world. You can borrow them, lean on them, and incorporate them into your own eating experiences. You can create your own practice. Explore your cultural heritage or the rituals of a culture you admire and bring a stress-free, mindful and healthy practice to your eating at any time. Throughout human history people have developed respectful ceremonies and rituals to acknowledge their appreciation for the food they eat and its source. You can explore these traditional pre-meal ceremonies and decide if a form of one will be helpful to you.

When Marcia began her eating disorder recovery efforts, she said, "I keep my journal. I see my therapist. I go to my support group. I'm learning to be kind and compassionate with myself. But I still panic around food. I don't know what to do. Please help me."

You may share her anguish and bewilderment as you struggle to develop more healthy attitudes about food and your eating habits.

Marcia, an agnostic wary of all things

religious or spiritual, created her own early pre-meal ritual. She said, "I dress nicely. I use a pretty plate and serve myself calmly at the table. I say to myself, 'I am nice.' I say to the food, 'You are nice.' And then I try to eat slowly."

This was her way of beginning. You can begin anyway you like.

The Judeo-Christian heritage offers an ancient ritual of saying grace before meals. You lower your head in respect to God and either fold your hands or hold hands with the people around you. You express your thanks to God and request to be worthy of God's gift of the food.

In the Hindu heritage, food is the physical manifestation of the supreme energy of the universe. A Sanskrit adage from Hindu tradition states "May the ones providing this food be happy and healthy."

Muslims say, "All praise is due to Allah who gave us food and drink and who made us Muslims."

Native Americans honor the positive qualities of the food source as they eat. For example, they express appreciation for the body and soul of the gifts given by the generosity of the corn or the sharp hearing of the rabbit.

Jews have prayers and blessings specific to

certain foods and have ritual handwashing as part of meal ceremonies. Before eating a meal that contains bread, they say, "Blessed are You, Lord, our God, King of the universe, Who brings forth bread from the earth."

A Buddhist pre-meal ritual statement, said aloud or silently, is:

"We receive this food in gratitude to all
    beings
Who have helped to bring it to our table,
And vow to respond in turn to those in
    need
With wisdom and compassion."

These pre-meal ceremonies may relate to God or spiritual forces in the universe or the power of life to sustain life. You can be of any heritage and faith (including atheist) and create a respectful pre-meal ceremony that is meaningful to you. Your ritual can give you an opportunity to experience peace with your food, a mindful attitude toward yourself, what you are about to eat, an appreciation for the forces that brought your food to you, and the people with whom you share your food.

Thousands of years ago, Buddhists developed a contemplative practice for eating called The Five Contemplations. Here is my edited version. I suggest that you refer to these contemplations often and continue them even when you are well into your recovery. They help you relate to food and eating with less stress. What's more, they may open your awareness to other aspects of your life that also need healing. They were written for people everywhere.

FIVE CONTEMPLATIONS WHILE EATING

1. I consider the work required in producing this food. I am grateful for its source.
2. I evaluate my virtues and examine any spiritual defects. The ratio between my virtues and defects determines how much I deserve this offering. (In other words, am I eating to exploit the food for emotional cravings and self-soothing, or am I eating for genuine life support and nourishment?)
3. I guard my heart cautiously from faults, particularly greed.
4. To strengthen and cure my weakening body, I consume this food as medicine.
5. As I continue on my spiritual or

healing path, I accept this offering with appreciation and gratitude.

I receive questions periodically about contemplation numbers two and three. As always, questions and comments inspire me to think, research, and write more. I found these contemplations written on the dining room wall in the Chinese Buddhist temple, Hsi Lai, in Hacienda Heights, California. Some of the phrasing and word choices may have been altered in translations from Chinese to English or from one time period to another.

First, these are contemplations, not rules. They are not meant to be followed like laws. They are meant to be considered at the most over a lifetime, and at the least, over the course of a meal. Different levels of meaning will occur to you over time if you continue to contemplate the words, thoughts, and feelings that come up.

Second, evaluating one's virtues and spiritual defects is a mighty challenge. Often, when you begin to explore your personal deficits, you can't think of a single one! Just as often, when you try to look deeply into the truth of who you are, you can't think of a single virtue either! What matters most is that you are looking. When you are more secure and capable of appraising yourself honestly and clearly, you discover character traits, good and not so good, that were invisible to you in the past. You become open to learning about yourself.

Openness, so different from secretiveness, allows you to see what you couldn't see, understand what you couldn't understand, forgive what you couldn't acknowledge. Your openness and willingness to explore your true nature allows you to give yourself compassion and the desire to care for your authentic self. You learn to appreciate the consequences of your actions and attitudes over a lifetime.

This contemplation allows you to open your heart and mind to the people around you, those who were around you in the past, and those who are yet to come into your life. You have an opportunity to become free as an imperfect being in an imperfect world where you are surrounded by imperfect others and can recognize, give, and receive love and respect.

This way of being in the world is very different from the life you lead with your eating disorder. Please remember, this is a glimpse of what can come for you in recovery. Contemplation and mindful practices, jibing and journaling, and mindful breathing and doing your affirmations gradually but inexorably will heal you and bring you health and freedom.

The act of eating embodies the giving and receiving of love and respect from one life form to another in order to maintain life on our planet. The contemplation of this statement can lead you to a new and profound wisdom.

So, starting from ignorance about your true self, how do you look at your defects and virtues? Because I was a visiting professional guest at the Sierra Tucson Eating Disorder Treatment Center in Arizona, I started receiving their alumnae newsletter, *Afterwords.* In the 2002–2003 Reunion issue, I came across an article by David Anderson, PhD. Dr. Anderson addresses the issues you and I are exploring together. He made a list combining the seven or eight deadly sins with ten personality disorders and came up with what he calls the "Eight Deadly Defects of Character":

1. Dishonesty/lack of authenticity/ wearing a "mask."
2. Pride/vanity/need for things to be "my way"/need to always be in control.
3. Pessimism/gloomy disposition/being

stuck in a "victim role." (This is closely associated with anger, bitterness, and resentment.)

4. Social, emotional, and spiritual isolation.
5. Sloth/laziness/passivity/living the unexamined life.
6. Gluttony/unwillingness to have self-discipline/a need for the quick fix.
7. Self-debasement/excessive self-denial and self-sacrifice.
8. Greed/lust/envy/materialism.

You can use his list as a starting place to consider what may apply to you (in different degrees at different times). Contemplation Two from Five Contemplations While Eating invites us to think about what virtues and defects are in ascendance at the moment. Many of these "defects" are actually symptoms of an eating disorder. Each will influence how you plan to eat, what and where you eat, how you relate to yourself and others while you eat, and how you think, feel, and communicate before, during, and after you eat.

A MINDFUL, HEALTHY, CARING APPROACH TO EATING

One way of eating involves receiving with grace, humility, respect, and gratitude an offering of life on the planet that nourishes your body and soul.

Hope, a fifty-three-year-old anthropologist, is doing research in Louisiana swamp country. She eats with care because she needs a strong healthy body that can endure the stress of heat, humidity, insect bites, and long waking hours.

Marcia, the graduate student, exchanged her chip eating ritual while studying for mindful meals at regular intervals when she discovered that she could read and absorb information for longer periods of time when she was well fed. To her surprise, she also discovered that instead of feeling stress because she stopped her mindless munching, she became more emotionally calm and secure because she was well nourished.

Grace, a thirty-eight-year-old new mother, ate with particular care despite her anorexia. She ate healthful foods because she was nursing her beloved baby girl. She wanted to give her baby the most nourishing milk her body could produce.

Florence, retired and a widow at eighty-three, eats thoughtfully and with care because she wants to be able to romp with her great-grandchildren for as long as possible.

What is your reason for wanting to eat well and be healthy? Journal about it and find your many answers.

Exploitative, Mindless, and Fear-Based Eating

Without realizing it, you may disregard the true meaning and value of food by exploiting it to manipulate or control your feelings.

Barbara, forty-five, married with a job and children, seemed to qualify for all eating disorder descriptions. She binged, purged, starved, overate, forgot to eat and had months at a stretch of eating normally. While in a normal eating phase, she went alone to visit her parents for their golden wedding anniversary. Family and friends gathered in an elegant restaurant known for quality gourmet food. Barbara ate what was offered, spoke charmingly with her parents and guests, and was gracious to strangers.

She left the party earlier than her parents because she wanted to be at their house alone. There she threw up, carefully identifying the partially digested or undigested foods that were pouring into the toilet. She

188

purged until her vomit was mixed with blood.

Barbara didn't know why she felt such urgency and determination to empty herself. She said she felt, after her purge, as if she had taken some kind of drug that made her feel as if she were asleep yet able to stand. She had nothing to say to her parents when they got home. They asked her if she felt all right because she looked like a zombie.

Barbara, in her dulled condition, had minimal awareness of herself or her parents. She thought nothing of the food she had eaten once she evacuated it. She only wanted to catch the next plane home.

To talk with Barbara about the value of the food she ate would be useless. She ate and purged in a mindless way out of fear she didn't even know she had. She had no ability to recognize what she ate as life being offered to her or to consider the plants and animals that became food for her, or the earth, rain, and sun that helped her food grow.

When Barbara negates her identity, her health, her very life and uses eating and purging to support that negation, she is also removing her appreciation of the life force of the food. Both she and the food become objects to use for emotional manipulations and control. She was not present enough to explore her defects or symptoms and consider the contemplations.

At home, feeling safe again, she returned to her breathing exercises and journaling. Backtracking from her episode at her parents' anniversary party, she discovered that she dreaded being with some of the family friends who were at the party and were very much a part of her childhood. She is gaining some understanding and compassion for herself and her fears.

Not eating also disregards the gifts of life. Claudia, twenty-seven but looking ancient and decrepit in her skeletal condition, refuses to eat. Despite her hunger pains, she enjoys feeling powerful when she looks at food but doesn't allow it in her body. She says she is reaching new spiritual highs by becoming as light as air. Yet she wastes food as her body wastes away. She uses self-sacrificial means to control others to make up for her lack of control in her life. She doesn't understand that she controls people by causing them worry and grief. She believes she is receiving adulation and deserving attention as others spend their time, money, and energy in their attempts keep her alive. Claudia, like Barbara, is lost in her eating disorder without knowing why. She is compelled to not eat just as Barbara was compelled to have her violent purge. Both are not able, yet, to benefit from wisdom that can emerge from addressing the contemplations. But, if she does the breathing, journaling and backtracking exercises consistently in a mindful way, eventually she will find her way to recovery.

These ancient contemplations are designed to increase your awareness and self-compassion. They help you dissolve your feelings of guilt and shame. When you binge or purge or starve or compulsively overeat, you can feel soul-eroding guilt and shame because you can't change your behavior.

Your guilt and shame come from a belief that you can control, through willpower, core emotions that are uncontrollable. This is why you also feel guilt and shame when your diets fail you.

The philosophy within the contemplations as well as your pre-meal rituals give you internal space to clear your guilt and shame and your belief in the power of your will. In the open place of calm and respect, you contemplate your behavior, your feelings, and your environment. You learn steadily, although perhaps imperceptibly, to be generous with yourself. You develop a generosity of spirit that allows you to open your mind and heart and ease the tension in your body. Without using willpower, you move toward your recovery naturally and organically at a pace that is right for you.

When you participate in pre-meal rituals and pay attention to ancient contemplations, without conscious effort you release yourself from stray remnants of the character defects on Dr. Anderson's list. When you remain aware of what nourishes life, you can appreciate that you are part of all life. You grow to understand that by living your life well you nourish yourself and others.

Then, as part of the joy of recovery, you live through your days, nights, meals, and snack times, not only with confidence and serenity, but with grace and a vibrant sense of well-being.

DAILY EXERCISES

1. Follow your breath for ten minutes at least three times a day.
2. Read or recite your three affirmations twenty times at least three times a day.
3. Copy the five contemplations, exploring whether any of the character traits or eating behaviors in this chapter ap-

ply to you.

4. Backtrack: Trace the source of the food you are about to eat before you eat it. Express your gratitude to the effort of everyone who contributed to the process that resulted in the food being before you now.

5. Experiment with pre-meal contemplations and rituals that might enrich your heart before you nourish your body.

CHAPTER 9
SPIRITUAL DEPTH

"The real voyage of discovery consists not in seeking new landscapes, but in having new eyes."
— Marcel Proust

What is spirituality, and how does it relate to your eating disorder? Exploring these questions and seeking answers that are right for you is part of your recovery work. An eating disorder gives you a seemingly reliable way to get and keep yourself out of trouble. When pain, anxiety, stress, too much excitement, fear, or despair come near, you turn to your eating disorder behaviors. They dull your sensitivity and give you a false sense of calm.

Often, women with eating disorders are described as having a waxy doll-like face. Unfortunately, in our culture, sometimes this is a compliment. Her face is doll-like because her facial muscles are not connected to her feelings. She is remote — not only from others but from herself. She is not attached to feelings she cannot bear to acknowledge.

However, the world is still functioning around her. Does this describe you? If you can't bear to take in negative information about your environment or the people in it, you are unaware of reality. This makes you more vulnerable and more likely to be a victim. Getting hurt physically or emotionally could jolt your false sense of equilibrium. You might wake up, but without recovery you will likely plunge into eating disorder behaviors.

Connecting with your spirituality is far more reliable and dependable than relying on your eating disorder. Personal spiritual depth helps you develop an inner strength that is more effective in coping with difficult feelings and situations. Rather than cause deficits in your life, spirituality gives you pleasure, richness, and appreciation for yourself, others, and the world.

Your eating disorder may wipe out your unwanted feelings if you can get the privacy and the right foods at the right time. You can reinforce your eating disorder "benefits" if you exercise yourself to exhaustion or have an emotional binge of rage at someone for their apparent transgressions. Your eating disorder demands a great deal from you in exchange for what it gives in return. You might want to journal on what your eating disorder demands of you in order for you to receive its "benefits." Here are a few:

- Isolation
- Poor health
- Poor teeth
- Loneliness
- Shame
- Fatigue

Some people avoid 12-step meetings because they think they would have to believe in God or because they can't accept a Higher Power, which they consider synonymous with God. Yet atheists and agnostics are part of all 12-step programs and stand alongside devout Catholics, Jews, or Evangelical Christians as they follow the recovery steps together.

This book is not a treatise on religions. Nor am I suggesting that you attend 12-step meetings. Only you can discover what is right and authentic for you. At the same time, I strongly encourage you to find a way to acknowledge your spiritual side and nurture it. It will help you meet your recovery challenges.

I was an active bingeing purging bulimic for twenty-nine years in a world where bulimia did not have a name. As my focused recovery unfolded I learned that, for me, spirituality means living a life of meaning. What is meaningful to you? Exploring this question can lead you to answers that heal your body and soul. I've found that my feelings of abandonment, isolation and worthlessness dissolved by living a life that is meaningful to me.

The experience of being grounded in a meaningful life evolves. It requires effort and appears in myriad forms for each person. Your goal is to be grounded. As you are more solidly present, what is meaningful to you becomes evident.

Meaning and purpose in life, based on a healing spirituality, can become integrated into your life over time through religion, spiritual practices, or good works. They can also come through commitment to an artistic endeavor — painting, sculpture, designing freeways, cleaning up a blighted area in town, or taking action to save the planet.

You can stumble into your authentic spiritual values through discoveries you make while taking actions that honor your heart. Mindfully raising a child, tending a garden or a store, teaching a class, or even cruising the Internet can be paths to spiritual depth.

Nora (not her real name) was my client so I heard the details of how she discovered her spiritual depth through cruising the Internet. She came to my private practice for psychotherapy to rid herself of her compulsive overeating. She was a talented and creative woman mired in, and seemingly committed to, an abusive work situation in the entertainment industry.

One night while surfing the Web she found a plea for medicine for children orphaned by AIDS in a developing country. Nora wrote to the organization and sent a check. The children's plight touched her heart and awakened a spiritual force she didn't know was within her. She rallied friends to contribute money to buy more medicine. Eventually, she brought groups of people to that country as volunteers to help build communities and escort large quantities of needed medicine to cities and towns in remote areas.

Sometimes men with guns confronted her and her guides. She used breathing exercises and affirmations as well as her growing courage and sturdy sense of commitment to weather these challenges. She brought children to the U.S. for medical attention. She contributed to girls learning to read and write in their country. She's not rich, but she's a happy woman, following where her heart leads. Each step deeper into her spiritual self gave her more strength and confidence. Her work inspired others, and they, in turn, inspired her with their help and commitment. This created an inner strength and sense of personal value far more sustaining than any eating disorder can offer.

Below are exercises that help you develop your path to your trustworthy and reliable spiritual force that will carry you through your life challenges. Use these exercises as you are ready to use them. Don't force yourself to do any. Don't judge yourself as you do the exercises you choose. The criteria for success only exist in your imagination. Let it go. Let yourself be open to surprise.

You can do one exercise many times or many one time. Some can be part of a daily or weekly practice. Some can be projects you take on for a limited time, the same as you might take on an eight- or ten-week class.

Still others might involve different kinds of commitment, such as learning and becoming proficient at a skill whether it is painting, karate, car racing, horseback riding, computer programming, debating, or learning to speak a new language. Others might surprise you by becoming part of your life journey forever.

I offer you what I hope are inspirational stories and ways to create your own path, but there is no map. You have openings in your heart and soul that yearn for fulfillment. Those are your beginning spiritual places. One step will lead to another.

Spirituality, as I use it here, is acknowledging, recognizing, respecting, and honoring your own essential life force within the context of the greater life force around you and in you. When you become more aware of your own essential nature, your awareness expands to acknowledge, recognize, respect, and honor the spirit of others. This awareness can keep expanding, as it does with the great spiritual beings of history, to include all living things.

Walking your personal spiritual path validates you and supports who you are and what you can be as you discover your potential. This is your core strength that makes the flimsy and destructive eating disorder you've relied on for so much of your life unnecessary.

What matters most is finding your path

and moving on it. In some ways we are always at the beginning wherever we are because we must always stay in the "now." The next moment hasn't happened yet, and so we are at the beginning in our efforts and in our recovery. This is good news because we can begin our recovery at any time.

I play a game in the car with my grand-daughters, at the time of this writing an impish bright-eyed three-year-old, Hannah, and a happy, mischievous and sturdy five-year-old, Delilah. As they ride in their car seats in the back of my Prius, I ask, "Where are you?" They shout, "We're here!" Then I say, "Where is that traffic light?" One or both will point and say, "It's over there." I ask, "Where are we going?" Delilah answers, "We're going there." I say, "Ah, but we can never get there." Hannah says, "Why? I can see it." Delilah says, "Oh yes, we can. We're going there right now."

I say, "You watch."

When we arrive at the traffic light, I ask, "Where are we?" If they say, "We're here!" I say, "Right." If they say, "We're there!" I say, "How can we be there if we are here?" "Where are we?" "Here!" they shout.

And so we drive, seeing all kinds of things out "there" and playing with the fact that we can never get "there." Yet all things come to us when we are "here." We have lots of giggles with this game. It's a kind of giggling spiritual practice.

Spiritual depth doesn't have to be serious, at least not all the time. It's about being present for what is. And the "what is" is the vastness of everything. We need to grow in our awareness to sense as much as we can, but never all of "what is." There's always more. We never run out. Beyond this planet is a solar system, and there are many solar systems in this universe. Through the warp and weave and black holes of space lie even more.

We begin with one tiny spot of here-and-now, and that is where you stand and see and smell and feel and taste in this particular moment. It's like your mindful exercise with the raisin, except now you are doing it with yourself and the immediate world around you.

The following exercises you can do at any time in any place. You can do them as first practices in developing your spiritual depth. You can do them for decades in the same way. The exercise doesn't change. You do.

1. NOTICING

- Be present for your feelings. Watch your breath and notice how your feelings move through you.
- Pay attention to what you are experiencing.
- Note what part of your experience is thinking.
- Note what part of your experience is emotion.
- Note what part of your experience is physical.

2. BODY SCAN

Lie down flat or with your legs raised on a pillow. Move your awareness slowly through your body, paying attention to large sections of yourself such as head, shoulders, torso, trunk, legs, feet, arms, and hands. You can do this in a more detailed way including skin, eyes, ears, nose, mouth, elbows, fingers, knees, ankles, and toes. You can be even more meticulous and include in your observation body organs, circulatory system, muscles, and nervous system. Depending on your time, inclination, and state of mind, choose the method that seems right for you now.

After you've done the body scan several times lying down, try it when you are sitting. When this is familiar to you, try it while walking. Eventually, you will be able to do this at any time, for example, on a bus, plane, or taxi; at your desk, walking to a meeting; waiting in line or for your children to finish their games; before you fall asleep at night or before you get out of bed in the morning.

Since you now know that your eating disorder blocks feelings, distorts perceptions and contributes to your harsh self-criticism, one recovery goal is to learn how to have an experience where you accept with no judgment at all. You've been doing the breath exercise. You are now more capable of patience. Your goal now is to come to your experiences as if you were brand new with no preconceived notions. You trust your ability to be present for whatever is happening in and around you. Eventually, you may find yourself laughing spontaneously. Your sense of humor can come to your aid. This is the experience of mindfulness and can lead you to clarity, freedom, self acceptance and a sense of being secure and grounded in the world.

I learned this for myself when I was visiting the island of Maui. Witnessing the sunrise over Haleakala was on my list of must dos. The concierge at my hotel told me it was a six-hour drive. I decided to make it a leisurely drive rather than a mission. I left my hotel before noon and drove through the island, stopping at beaches, shops, and garage sales as I meandered toward the volcano. I was enjoying myself, and time rolled on.

When I got to the slope, it was much later than my schedule allowed. Still, I thought I could make it by sunrise. I neglected to factor in the unlighted, narrow twisting road that forced me to drive slowly and cautiously. I had been so intent on seeing the sunrise I had forgotten about darkness and night.

The stars came out. I couldn't see the vistas below me as I climbed the mountain, but I could feel vast space growing and stretching over the cliff edge beyond my little road. Sometimes I stopped at a turnout on the mountainside to see the dark sky and sparkling stars and to hear the wondrous silence.

About a half-hour before sunrise, according to my calculations, the dark around me got darker still. Starlight was gone. I stopped the car, turned off the lights, and put my hand in front of my face. I couldn't see it. It was that dark.

The cliché, "It's always darkest before the dawn," occurred to me.

That wasn't a metaphor at all! It was true. I felt a surge of comfort that softened my face into a smile and warmed my shoulders and my chest from the inside. I felt that I was on to something and that I was in the right place at the right time doing the right thing for reasons beyond my knowing.

I reached the top of the mountain and parked my car. I found a huge boulder overlooking the miles of open crater that I couldn't yet see in the dim light. I leaned into the boulder, wiggled my body until I found my "spot," and waited in my ringside seat for the show.

It didn't happen. Ten, fifteen, twenty minutes, and it didn't happen. I got impatient. Where was it? How long does a sunrise take? I got here on time. Where are you?

I waited. I could feel tension coming up in my chest. The warmth of my smile was gone. I wanted the spectacle of sunrise at Haleakala now!

Then I had the insight that will last me a lifetime. This was not a TV program nor did I get to turn the on/off switch. This wasn't a movie with a specific start time. This was sunrise at Haleakala — God's time!

God's time? Of course. I felt sheepish and forgiven at the same time.

All my plans, preconceptions, rules, expectations, judgments, demands, and feelings of entitlement dissolved in that term, "God's time." I breathed more easily. The boulder behind my back was my home and my friend. It was created in God's time, so was I and so was the ground I stood on. I looked at the faint tint of color in the sky. I heard the birds' early morning songs. I saw a few other people in the distance, standing like quiet sentries sharing this moment.

God's time, this time, past time, coming time — God's time, not mine. But I was part of God's time. And the sun did rise. And the colors rolled gently like a wave over that vast expanse. It left a permanent picture in my mind's eye and a permanent appreciation of letting go and being present for more than I could imagine.

What's more, I felt a greater liking for myself. This was more than self-confidence, although that was part of it. I knew that coming here was important for me to do, even though I hadn't known why. Somehow, as part of God's time, I experimented with time to get here. I calculated and strategized and made my decision, based on a goal I only dimly appreciated. I wondered about those stops I made along the way. If I had stopped more or less frequently would I have had the experience I had?

There's no reasonable answer to this question, but in my heart I felt and still feel that I was connected with something bigger than me in ways that I didn't, and couldn't, know. A cooperative effort was going on that made this experience come out for me in the wonderful way it did. What's more, I believe that many of those other people, those sentries on alert who also responded to the call of sunrise at Haleakala, had their own experiences, different from mine but equally or perhaps even more profound. I felt kindly toward all of them. Kindly. The word must be connected to the word kinship.

What we do as individuals to achieve spiritual depth we can do as groups and even nations and perhaps as a world community. We are, after all, individual human beings. We all breathe. We all were born, and we all will die. Yet some of us sing. Some of us inspire each other. How far can it go, this inspiration — this giving of the breath of life?

It begins on an individual basis. You. Me. And then, us.

First you heal and develop beyond the limits enforced by your eating disorder. As your way of being in the world shifts, based on what you discover in these simple exercises, your responses to situations and other people change. Your decision-making process changes. You say yes and no differently, and ultimately that changes your environment and your life.

Other people will notice. You will notice them noticing you. A new kind of awareness begins and expands to include more people. Most of us are grateful to have a channel through which to share stories and feelings and take action on our heartfelt desires. When you are more present, you take in and are aware of life in a far-reaching way. When you touch another healthy person with your awareness and presence, they feel included, expanding in their own awareness to reciprocate.

I say healthy people, because some frightened and limited people do not want to be known or, for that matter, even know themselves.

A lovely woman, Roberta, as part of her therapy for bulimia, worked through her difficulties in drawing boundaries with me. One evening she attended a professional social gathering at UCLA. A male colleague she knew slightly stood in a small circle of people when she joined them. During the hellos, he stepped eagerly toward her with his arms outstretched for a full body hug. She stepped back firmly and stretched out her arm to shake hands and to keep him at his distance. He stopped, startled, and shook her hand. She remained engaged with the people in the circle. She said she felt that the men looked at her with new respect.

Later in the evening several women colleagues approached her and asked, "How did you do that?" The invasive man was in the habit of getting full body hugs from his professional colleagues who were unwilling but who didn't want to make a scene. Roberta realized she responded differently on this occasion because she had incorporated her awareness exercises with her authentic values. She drew on internal resources she didn't know she had, but which now came to her in a natural way. She saw that the other women knew what was pleasant and unpleasant. But they couldn't gather themselves into an integrated whole with the sturdiness of spirit to risk disrupting a professional gathering and honoring their self-respect.

Roberta was happily surprised to discover her spirituality practices could have such a concrete and practical effect in her life. She also acquired a more positive reputation with her colleagues.

Without intending to, Roberta helped others to move toward greater self-respect and courage through a brief but influential moment in her life. She made a quick scan of her comfort, neutral, and discomfort areas with lightning speed, made her decision and commitment, stepped back and held out her hand. By so doing, she inspired something beyond her own immediate experience and was instrumental in expanding the awareness and courage of others.

You can't look after others well until you can look after yourself. Expecting someone to care for you because you care for them is bargain-based. You place a value on what you give, and you expect equal reciprocity. That's not spirituality. Being present and authentic for yourself allows you to be present and authentic for others — and they you. In that genuine connection, something wonderful can happen. Spirituality is not bargain based.

Rachel had eaten compulsively since she was fifteen. Now, at fifty-six, with a quick-tempered husband and a bi-polar adult son living at home, she struggled for peace by making unwelcome demands on her family. Out of desperation and with little faith that she would find help, she began daily mindfulness practices. She did either a body scan or her breathing exercise every morning. After a month of this she said, "Something is different. I don't know how it happened. Bill (her husband) isn't fighting with me. Tommy (her son) wants me to call him Tom and hung up his clothes himself for the first time since I don't remember when."

We acknowledged this change but did not explore it. She didn't yet realize that integrating herself in a new way evoked a different response from the two men in her life.

After ten more weeks passed, she described a "fun lunch" she had with Tom at a café. They were making plans for him to be alone for the weekend while she and Bill took a little "get away" vacation nearby.

I commented on the positive changes in her family life and asked her what she supposed was going on.

Rachel said, "You're right. Bill and Tom are much easier to get along with." As we explored, she said, "When I first did my mindfulness exercises I was bored and restless. But you said to keep doing them anyway, so I did. I was actually a little mad at you about that. But I kept doing them.

"Then I started to like doing them. I felt smaller than what I thought I was and bigger at the same time. Does that make sense? I felt like I was a different person but more like me too. After a couple of months I started to have those feelings when I wasn't doing the exercises."

I asked her if she could tell me the difference between what a normal day was for her before she did the mindfulness practices and what a normal day was for her now.

She thought for a moment and said with some surprise, "My days are really different. I wake up earlier than Bill now and do my exercises while he is asleep.

"Then I make breakfast and read the paper. Bill likes to smell coffee when he wakes up, and he likes not having to get the paper. We talk in the mornings now before he goes to work.

"Because the exercises take up time, I don't go in Tom's room in the morning to check on him and ask him to clean up his room or get ready for his part time job. He was angry at me the first week, but then he started getting up on his own. He liked finding coffee ready too, and he started making his own breakfast.

"Oh, by the way. Did I tell you I lost five pounds?"

The beauty of mindfulness practice is that many positive benefits evolve naturally as you drop control and judgment and pay precise attention to yourself and your environment. Rachel gave up doing some caretaking chores for Bill and Tom, chores she felt were burdensome, and she gave up her feeling of being owed payment. She was coming together as the woman she authentically is. That gave her freedom and clarity to appreciate what was meaningful in her life and to discard what was not. Her growing satisfaction in her ordinary day created a ripple effect that inspired her family.

Rachel let go of how she thought her husband and son should behave. She let go of how she should look or what kind of treatment her family owed her. She liked her mindfulness practices because she discovered she had expectations that were artificial and controlling, and she decided they were just silly. She then discovered that without those expectations she could see what was lovely in her life or what could be lovely if she gave herself the attention she needed.

As she lived this out by following her heart and letting Bill and Tom deal with it, she disrupted the family routine. Once Bill and Tom realized that this was a permanent change, they adapted. Bill enjoyed Rachel because she was less tense and more his friend again. Tom liked being called by a more adult name and being treated more like an adult. He felt Rachel's lack of demands was a sign of respect to him, and he wanted to live up to the good feelings that were building in him.

These positive changes in behavior and feelings grow exponentially once they begin because everyone is being more appreciative and open with everyone else. Their lives together and separately blossom. Rachel doesn't know how she lost the five pounds. She's not counting calories. She is not eating compulsively. She is unaware of how her more expanded and clear way of being in the world makes her compulsive overeating unnecessary.

I encourage you to be aware of Rachel's process and pay attention to the details in your life. It seems that nothing is of no consequence. Everything counts. Each chapter in this book is ostensibly about a different topic, yet all the topics are part of the framework of your experience. The exercises throughout this book, and more vividly in this chapter, give direct attention to a healing and integration process that is so necessary for you to be present and honor the authentic woman you are. When you appreciate and can rejoice in your own authenticity you have no need for an eating disorder or any other toxic influence in your life.

The exercises and activities are simple. They don't seem directly related to your specific difficulties or challenges, yet they are the core of what can unite you into a harmonious whole.

If you are divided inside and using your eating disorder to prevent yourself from knowing who and even where you are, then you cannot imagine inner wholeness and integration. Your eating disorder creates perceptual distortions so your evaluations are often not relevant to your making genuine and helpful behavorial changes. You need to be aware and present.

Once you are on your recovery path, you will recognize other people who are also recovering. When your healing energy gathers in you, it shows in your face, your voice, and your actions. As Rachel continued to become more whole, she laughed and said, "My neighbor asked me if I had a facial. My mother asked me if I changed my hair. My girlfriend asked me if I was having an affair. My women's club wants me to run for an office." She added, "I think we're on to something!"

In recovery you know when to reach out and help someone, and you are more open to others reaching out to help you. Plus, you know the difference between exploitation based on your weaknesses and support based on your healthy pursuits that need a loving "boost" now and then.

The exercises in this book help you cope with a given situation and teach you new options, strengthen you to say no to what you don't want, and give power to the yes that leads you to your authentic goals. Try the basic exercises at the end of each chapter or see additional exercises in Appendix B to find what seems right for you in any phase of your recovery.

Living with an eating disorder stops you from knowing you have a storm of powerful energies crashing within you and over which you have no control. All you can do is scramble to block out your awareness to get relief. Your inner storm remains and may require more eating disorder behaviors to keep your blocks to awareness in place.

When you acknowledge the storm, you can pay attention, rally your strength and resources, and work to care for yourself in a realistic way. You even find ways to make the storm's energy work for you. It's your energy. If you are more whole and sturdy yourself you channel that energy into a project you care about.

After three years of recovery work Dee Dee stopped wishing about her career in music that she had dreamed of all her life and started putting energy into making it happen. She took guitar lessons and practiced regularly. She joined music groups where musicians met to play with one another and comment on style and choices. She took a class in music for films. She plays guitar in little theater productions now and is optimistic about what might come next for her.

Keira, recovering from anorexia, discovered that some of her fears, though vivid, were as fake as a hologram and had no substance. On the phone, her mother said, "I'll tell you what your sister did, but promise not to tell her I told you." Keira was frightened to disobey her mother, the woman she loved but who punished her severely as a child and locked her in closets for disobedience. Keira did a quick breathing exercise, did a quick body scan of her thumping heart, and said, "If it's a secret, don't tell me. I won't keep a secret."

She kept doing mindful breathing while she waited for the explosion. Her mother was silent for a moment and then said, "Oh well, I'll tell you anyway," and went on. Keira was flabbergasted at the simplicity and immediate success of her revolutionary act. She said, "I was afraid to go against my mother's wishes for years. And I had nothing to be afraid of. I could have set myself free any time." But she needed to be in recovery to know that.

Alternatively, you may discover that your fears are based on genuine and imminent danger that must be addressed immediately. If you are obsessed with your food and weight, you distract your attention from what is going on around you.

Melinda, reluctantly and with much support, began doing some of the exercises in this book. She couldn't do them on her own because of the severity of her fears and food cravings. So she joined meditation and mindfulness groups and listened to mindfulness and meditation tapes and CDs. As she became more aware, she became more frightened. She needed more support and more appointments with me to tolerate her fears without resorting to binge/purge episodes or dropping weight to dangerous levels.

Eventually, her fog lifted and clarity emerged. Her husband was gay and had been having anonymous sexual encounters with men. Their finances were in ruins.

Melinda's personal growth and healing equipped her to reach a level of internal sturdiness and faith in herself so she could allow herself to recognize her reality, rather than experience those clues as triggers for her eating disorder. While the information was terrible, knowing the truth gave her an opportunity to make decisions and take actions that were far more helpful than eating a half gallon of ice cream in front of the TV.

In recovery you replace your eating disorder with awareness and courage so you live well in a way that is fulfilling for you.

Even now, regardless of how you feel in this moment, if you are reading this and working toward your recovery, you are not overwhelmed. You are building what you need to create and nurture your ability to be present. Your experience of being fully present will give you clarity and the courage to make wise decisions.

How can you step to the side of your anxious, fearful, angry, or impatient reactions and free your life force? It's simple. Not easy, but simple. When faced with a challenging situation, use your breathing exercise. Give your mind freedom to allow your intelligence, creativity, emotions, and authentic values to come together to alert you to a possible solution. You can do your breathing exercise in the shower or before you put on your shoes, walk through a doorway, start the car, put the children to bed, greet your guests, or pick up the phone.

Use any mindful practice in this book before you commit to a decision to take action, whether it be writing an emotionally charged letter or e-mail, or starting or ending a relationship. You could be unaware that you are about to act impulsively based on mindlessness or fear. Pausing or taking a fifteen-minute break or giving yourself a day or two to mindfully breathe, do a body scan, or journal may alert you to issues you didn't see and ground you in the reality of here and now.

The nice thing about the breathing exercise is that it's invisible. It requires no sound, no words, no props, or particular positions that would attract attention. You can do it in waiting rooms, on hold, or while waiting for your lunch date.

As you do your exercises, your own spiritual beliefs will become clearer to you. You may find that they bring you "home" to the religion or spiritual practices of your heritage or of your childhood. You may discover that your favorite books, films, and poems reveal a spiritual theme that you yearned for but never believed could be yours. You reveal your own spirituality to yourself in freedom.

With courage and presence, you can trust your spirituality to lead you to a more authentic way of being in this world — a way that is more reliable and sturdy than your eating disorder could ever offer.

When you use your strength, courage, and commitment to follow your heart, you are on your spiritual path. You become the heroine in your life story. Spiritual depth supports heroines on their recovery journey when they face their great terrors. It helps you face terror and evokes personal wisdom.

You may not ever have to face threatening guards who point loaded weapons at you while you travel your path, vulnerable in remote regions of a developing country. You will, however, need to face and cope with your inner terrors that fill you with a sense of desolation and helplessness. We all do. With every step of your recovery path, you learn to use your eating disorder less and your inner strength and wisdom more.

If you are not present and aware in this real and flawed world, you not only limit your understanding of what is, but you fill in blanks with your fantasies. You live a life based on what you prefer to see, as Melinda did by not recognizing the sexual orientation of her husband or the real state of their finances. The manufactured "pretend world" you prefer to believe in puts you in danger. You might protect yourself from feeling grief, loss, or horror if you are hiding from the knowledge that you are dependent on an abuser or exploiter. But you do nothing to protect yourself from being dependent on a dangerous person.

To keep your awareness at bay, you need your eating disorder and perhaps other aids like drugs or alcohol to drown your senses. Too much or too little food or sleep will help by dulling your mind and distorting your thoughts. You may need extra pounds of weight to buffer you or an obsession with thinness that cannot be achieved to distract you from knowledge of your own life situation.

Simply dropping your eating disorder behavior, as if you could, only exposes your hidden fears and vulnerabilities. You need to be able to tolerate what you experience in life without using your eating disorder in order to be truly free. That means you continually work to clear your mind, give up judgment and control, and learn to say no in a meaningful way. You build your strength, skills, and resources to face in the here and now what you couldn't face in the past.

This is the greatest challenge in eating disorder recovery. To be realistic and present requires letting go of cherished illusions. Your practices are helping you to build and develop from within so you can move through your imaginary and real "dark nights of the soul" and come through to a healthy and free new morning.

DAILY EXERCISES

1. Follow your breath for ten minutes at least three times a day.
2. Read or recite your three affirmations twenty times at least three times a day.
3. Do a full body scan at least three times a week.
4. Write about what sacred means to you. Ask the page, "How will I know what is sacred to me? How will I honor that?" Write the answers that come to you. Draw no quick conclusions. Keep writing and asking. Over time you will see themes that lead to

the sacred places within you.

5. Backtrack: Regardless of your beliefs today, explore and learn about the beliefs of your parents and grand-parents. Go further back if you can to the spiritual beliefs of the ancestors that created your heritage.

CHAPTER 10
THE GREAT TERROR

"In a real dark night of the soul, it is always three o'clock in the morning. . . ."
— F. Scott Fitzgerald

At some point in your recovery work, the feelings your eating disorder covers will come roaring up, leaving you terrified. It's only fair to let you know this. You might think you are going crazy, but please know that you are not. You are releasing a torrent of blocked emotions.

You know how entrenched your eating disorder has been in your life. It has protected you from feelings you could not bear. Now you are growing strong and resilient. You are developing courage. You need it all to cope with your feelings without using your eating disorder. When these feelings erupt, you experience your dark night of the soul.

In daylight hours when you are in this

fear, you might distract yourself by activity, companionship, or thinking about the plight of people in more devastating circumstances. But these distractions won't give you respite at three o'clock in the morning.

Alone, or feeling alone, and surrounded by darkness, when your deep fears rise you don't know the difference between reality and fantasy. Your shaking body is real. Your fear is real, but you don't know what else might be real. Is the source of your fear a real threat in the present, or is it a memory from the past, or a delusion stemming from extreme loneliness and loss of self-confidence? Is it better to escape from your fear in whatever way you can, or is it better to confront it? If you confront it, will it destroy you, or will you find relief? If you share it, will you be punished or ridiculed? If you hide under the covers, can you wait until your fear goes away? Will they go away?

In the midst of your terror, you might fake competence and respond to a knock on the door, a phone call, or a hungry child. You deal with the reality as quickly as you can so you can return to what is truly real for you — your terror. You are compelled to remain there and hope that the darkness will lift by some magical force, yet, as you wait, you feel the essence of your identity fade. You want to be saved, but you are certain nothing can save you.

This terror marks the boundary between your living a life with an eating disorder or living in recovery. Meeting this challenge and crossing the threshold to what lies beyond your terror is your route to freedom. You have been equipping yourself all along to be capable of meeting this challenge. As much as you'd like to get it over with, you will not cross this threshold easily or quickly. Your first step toward success is to feel these feelings and know, while you are feeling them, that you are not crazy and that this is part of your recovery work.

What's happening is that you dropped through your adult façade and your adult resources into your undeveloped child psyche. You are a motherless child alone in the dark. You may have catastrophic thoughts, the equivalent of a child's night terrors, awake or asleep. In this state your mind will create exaggerated horrors to match your feelings. Even the worst fantasies are more tolerable than what feels like endless fear.

Marilyn, forty-seven, divorced, and on her own for five years, would swing between anorexia and bulimia. She was in the first six months of her recovery work when her great terror hit. She was home alone, hiding under the covers in bed, eating fast from a large bag of cookies. Still eating, she got up and paced through the house seeing vivid colors through a haze. She was afraid of her furniture and couldn't bear to look out a window. She turned on the television but couldn't sit still to watch it. She saw her bag of cookies was empty, dropped the bag on the floor, and got a box of cereal from her kitchen cupboard. She returned to the TV, eating handfuls of cereal out of the box while she changed channels fast. She was looking for a program that would take her out of herself. Her phone rang. She jumped in fear, watched the phone till it stopped ringing. She couldn't pick it up. She paced and ate, trembled and cried — and didn't know why.

Trisha, also forty-seven and in the early stages of bulimia recovery, got hit with her terror and couldn't bear to be alone. She got in her car and sped down the freeway alternating between screaming and eating from a large box of doughnuts on the passenger seat. She was on her way to have sex with a man she didn't like because she called him and he said, "come over."

How do *you* respond to terror? Do you cower in a corner not wanting anyone to see you? Do you grab on to anything or anyone that you hope will soothe you? Do you binge or purge? Do you run on the treadmill until you are exhausted?

When you are in the grip of your frightened undeveloped child psyche, the adult in you is not available. You have no mature options so your terrors escalate.

When your terror episode passes (and it does pass), you don't return to your life unharmed. Both Marilyn and Trisha ate too much and overloaded on sugar. Maybe the phone call that Marilyn didn't answer was important. Trisha could have had an automobile accident or been stopped by the police or had a sexual experience that pulled her into an unsavory situation. Marilyn's terror episode lasted four days and nights. She didn't go out. She threw up often. She thought about suicide and frightened herself more.

Trisha came home from her sexual experience feeling ashamed and unclean. Instead of getting relief and a budding sense of self confidence, she felt unlovable, unworthy, and in greater despair. She binged more on doughnuts until she slept as if she had knocked herself unconscious.

You don't have to live a story like this. You can answer your own 911 call. This is vital to your recovery work.

When you are in torment, please know that, as horrible as it is, you are exposing a wound that needs healing. You are in the midst of a painful opportunity to discover and apply what your heart and soul need to heal.

This brush with your dark night of the soul is a long honored human experience. The term is not just poetry. Religions around the world describe this feeling of desolation, fear, and despair. Søren Kierkegaard, the famous Danish philosopher, titled one of his most acclaimed books, *Fear and Trembling,* from the New Testament reference to Philippians 2:12, ". . . continue to work out your salvation with fear and trembling."

How might you approach your own self when your terror descends? First, you might try to talk yourself out of your fear by saying, "Nothing really bad is happening right now," but that doesn't work because your body is trembling and fear permeates your entire experience, making even familiar objects seem alien and strange. You feel you don't belong anywhere.

You try to escape into a movie or a binge or treadmill or pills or alcohol, but you either get no relief or the relief is short lived.

You curl up into a corner of your bed or couch and bury yourself under a blanket. When someone attempts to contact you or you look at your mail, a newspaper, or a task still undone, you feel more frightened.

Responding to a call or seeing tasks or even reading material designed for an adult brings up more anxiety.

Your terror grows as you discover your feeble attempt to escape did not work and will not work. You rush to what gave you respite in the past. You hope you can "go away" long enough so that when you "return" your terror is over. But if you are "gone" long enough, it's not the terror that disappears, but you, as your own personality disintegrates.

You've got to find a way to be "here" when this is the last place you want to be. The longer you escape fears using your eating disorder, the stronger your fears will become. You need firm boundaries to contain them and you have none. If you are not "here" your fears will flood your present leaving you only "there" to be safe and "there" is pure fantasy.

When you are in your normal functioning life, your terrors seem far away, almost as if they didn't exist, but when they come back, they come hard. Your denial that kept your terror away from your awareness betrays you. Fear floods you again. When it's overwhelming, you don't know how to think about it because you can't think. You want to hang on to something. Because you don't know what will save you, you'll grab on to anything — like doughnuts or a package of cereal or a dark corner of your couch.

Your terror is a healing crisis. You can't let anyone see you or be with you because you believe you are too horrible in this condition for anyone to tolerate. If you do call for help, you can't accept it. You counter every positive possibility with a sincere and agonizing no. You are lost, and you know it. Discovering who and what you can trust that might be helpful to you in your crisis is a major victory in crossing the threshold into your recovery.

Your collapsed denial that opens the gates to your fears is opportunity. You knew you didn't want to feel your feelings, but you had no idea how deep and strong these feelings went. Your terror teaches you why you need your eating disorder. There are voids in your psychological development that you fall into if you don't use your eating disorder to fill in your gaps. Your terror is so inescapable that you choose your eating disorder every time you have a choice. This is why you gain back weight. This is why diets fail. This is what needs to be addressed for you to be sturdy in recovery.

In an unguarded moment your defense system fails to block what triggers your fear. That means your system for taking care of yourself has flaws. As you age, your life gets more complex. You have more responsibilities. You have more challenges in an adult world.

You developed your methods of defending yourself when you were young — at whatever age you were when the earliest traces of your eating disorder began. Your system is geared to defend you against the challenges you faced as a child.

Now you are expected to meet the world as a competent and functioning adult. Your defense system is not sophisticated enough or fine tuned enough to work well in adult society. When your defenses collapse under adult expectations, you find yourself cast into the all too familiar zone of terror. Your wounded and immature part of your psyche cannot cope.

But there's more to you than that part. You need to bring your adult presence to the frightened aspect of your own heart and soul. This is why I've been giving you your breathing exercises, your body scan instructions, your journaling, affirmations and backtracking practices. You have been building strength, wisdom, compassion and courage to bring to this frightened and abandoned part of your own self.

Terror is your signal. Your heart is calling 911. Here's how you start to rescue yourself. First, know that you are in this terror again. You've been here before and came out of it. Hang on to that thought as you grope your way to what will ground you.

Write down what you are feeling. Just keep writing. That is a lifeline that can pull you out of raging waters. Describe your body sensations. Describe how the room looks to you. Scream on the page everything you want to scream aloud. Keep writing lists of what you like and don't like about yourself, about other people, about your home, your neighborhood, your job, or your school. Make lists of what you have that's good and what you want. Keep writing. Describe how the pen feels in your hand and what the paper looks like. Keep writing. Writing is grounding. Writing will help you connect with gravity again.

You need to know that you are not alone and that someone understands you. Go to your poetry books or go online to a poetry site. Keep looking at poems until you find one that describes what you are feeling. Those poems are there. What you feel is part of the human condition. Great suffering reveals the human condition. Maybe find Shakespeare. Maybe Yeats. Maybe Poe. Maybe "Invictus" speaks to you or Vachel Lindsay. F. Scott Fitzgerald knows about these feelings and so does *The Bell Jar* author Sylvia Plath. You need to be close to words that describe tragedy or rage or fear or deep sorrow. You can find them. They will match your experience, and you will feel part of the human race again.

You may need gentle soothing and holding or to be rocked like a child. You can watch children's programming: *Little Bear, Caillou, Madeline, Clifford the Big Red Dog, Teletubbies.* Hold a teddy bear or a pillow and sink yourself into the sweetness of stories that are full of love, honesty, caring, and health. There's a part of you that needs these stories now. This is not falling into meaningless fantasy. This is meeting the needs of your undeveloped psyche. You can nourish "little you" gently and with love as you give yourself what you need to grow toward a more mature state. Don't hide or punish that frightened aspect of yourself. Thoughtfully love that part of you all the way up to competent adulthood where the small frightened aspect of you can bring her gifts to the whole that is you.

If you are capable of reading in your frightened state, reach for the old classic unabridged fairy tales. Read them. True fairy tales begin with something out of balance. The king or queen is dead. Famine is on the land. A dragon or giant or evil spell is causing hardship to individuals or the entire kingdom. The fairy tale progresses through various challenges until the story reaches its happily-ever-after ending. That ending is always a healing of the original problem. The fractured state at the beginning achieves wholeness. Reading these stories, especially when you are in the dark of your darkest times, will allow small and large parts of your psyche to grab hold of the healing momentum within the story and discover their own ways of seeking integration. This leads to your wholeness. You do not need to be consciously aware of this process. You just have to supply the nourishment you need. Your psyche will take it, and you'll heal.

Read Joseph Campbell's *The Hero with a Thousand Faces*. If you look carefully, you will see that you, too, are a heroine moving through a classic human story. Don't forget *The Baby-sitters Club* series by Ann M. Martin. I keep an ample supply of these books on hand to give to clients. These stories brilliantly address the needs and challenges of young teenage girls. If your eating disorder began in your teens, your psychological development stopped in your teens. You've been caring for yourself with your eating disorder, and the genuine care you needed as a teen never got through. Martin's books go straight to that naïve, unprotected, and unaware adolescent in your heart. Cherish yourself and let Martin help you develop so your fears don't overwhelm you anymore.

Great art is also a recovery tool. If your terror is too great for you to drive or even walk, have a friend take you to a museum, or if you have access to art books at home, scan through art the same way you scanned through poetry. You can go to any museum in the world via the Internet now. You can visit the Louvre. Someone has painted or sculpted what you are feeling. Get as close to that art as you can. You will be able to breathe again as your psyche meets a consciousness that understands.

You can even learn from classic detective stories. The determined detective hero represents light and health as he seeks out the dark villain, sorts out chaos, and establishes health, equilibrium, and safety.

You can cast runes and address the I Ching; ask questions, ask for help. Allow the coins and glyphs to take you to positive thoughts that are not accessible to your own mind right now. This is also a way of connecting with wise words and caring ideas that are simply not available to you while you are in your terror state. You can hold on to caring wisdom until your terror wave passes and you can sleep.

You can also call a 12-step hotline. Whether or not you attend meetings, program people will accept your call. You can speak with a person in recovery. Anyone in genuine recovery knows about the dark night of the soul. A hotline counselor can meet you where you are and listen. The presence of another living voice that can be with you will help you ride out your storm. In that conversation, you can speak as you would to a page in your journal; the talk, as the writing, will help you endure and explore what you feel.

A major benefit in following these suggestions is that when your terror episode passes, you know you survived. Not only did you survive, but you didn't cause any damage to yourself or anyone else. When you came out of it, you came back unharmed to your world. This knowledge about yourself and your accomplishment enlightens and strengthens you.

Your path to recovery doesn't sidestep terror episodes. You may want to skip them. I don't blame you. But the terror place is there. You need to learn ways that make that place much smaller and less frightening and yourself more capable.

Eating disorder recovery doesn't mean moving to a trouble-free life of sustained good feelings, normal eating, and an attractive body. Eating disorder recovery means that you are healthy, strong, resilient, creative, and mature so that you can cope and deal with what reality brings to you. You stay conscious. You stay present. You gather your resources and expand them to cope well and live. Your increased maturity and health, and better access to your authentic mind and spiritual depth, will see you through.

DAILY EXERCISES

1. Follow your breath for ten minutes at least three times a day.
2. Read or recite your three affirmations twenty times at least three times a day.
3. Journal: As part of your journaling,

explore your childhood fears. What occasions do you remember when you were afraid. What care and comforting reassured you? In your journal describe yourself as a child in fear. Then, as the adult you are now, join the child on the page, giving her what she needs. Ask on the page, "How can I get to know you and be your helpful adult friend? Write the answers that come to you.

4. Backtrack the experience that helped you sustain yourself during your terror. If it was a poem, backtrack the poem through books, performances, schools. Go further back and explore what was going on in the author's life at the time he or she wrote the poem. Do the same if it was a work of art or ancient words of wisdom. Backtrack the present day hotline counselor — who is she, where did she come from, how did she happen to answer the phone?

CHAPTER 11
RECOVERY CHECK-IN

"I do not understand the mystery of grace
— only that it meets us where we are and
does not leave us where it found us."
— Anne Lamott

By reading this book and following suggestions that seem relevant for your recovery, you've been having powerful emotional experiences and making changes in your life. Before we go further, take a look at how you are doing. Eating disorders play havoc with your digestion. In recovery your body learns to digest. Your mind and spirit also need time to digest the new recovery information and skills you are feeding yourself.

Have your daily, weekly, and monthly activities and routines changed at all? What have you stopped? What have you begun? What's different in your perceptions? Do you notice any change in how you respond to people or how they respond to you?

Here is a recovery check-in dream. Julie is a fifty-three-year-old woman with ten years of recovery from bulimia and binge eating. She has a delightful family, is a successful artist, and is financially well rewarded for her work. She feels free from her eating disorder behaviors. Sometimes, however, she feels the old cravings when she is about to stretch beyond her familiar routine into a new creative endeavor. She had this dream as she was starting a new series of paintings, the biggest and most lucrative commission of her career.

Julie dreamed that a living baby in a plastic bag was placed, as a joke, next to a murdered baby, dead for over forty years. In her dream she shouted, "What do you think you are doing? This is a baby, a human being!"

The jokester, an unkempt man, laughed. Julie shouted again, "You are torturing this baby. You put it in a plastic bag. You laid it next to a corpse. How would you feel if someone did that to you? How would you feel, helpless, imprisoned, ignored, and lying next to a corpse? How would you like to be abandoned, made a joke of, and laid next to a murder victim, maybe feeling certain that this was to be your fate too?"

The jokester was stunned. He said, "Babies don't feel stuff like that."

Julie said, "Of course they do. This is a little human being!"

She then noticed her childhood friends and family at the scene. They stared at her as if she were a strange "thing" in their midst. Julie wanted to take off all her clothes and go naked into the snow to show them how stripped and exposed she felt. But she didn't. She took the baby, pulled off the plastic, covered the infant with her new warm coat and walked away. She knew this was a permanent end to any contact with these people.

When Julie awoke and wrote down her dream, she realized how true it was. Her need to separate from her former way of living was real, although not so vivid and dramatic as in her dream.

Her eating disorder numbed her to the torment in her childhood. As she grew, she worked her way through dangerous relationships, brushes with the law, and failed attempts at getting an education until she found recovery. She separated from negativity as she built a new life based on the authentic values she discovered in herself as her health improved. She found a career, made a family, developed friends, became financially stable. She didn't throw up. She didn't binge. She rarely overate for emotional reasons.

The first baby in her dream, representing her beginning in life, was killed off early. Now, many years later that murder is exposed. Vulnerable new life comes again as she finds her way to recovery, her art, and loving relationships. However, lurking ignorance is ready to tease and traumatize the new life to death. Julie, now aware, recognizes the danger, and her protective passions are aroused. She rushes in outrage to rescue and free the living baby, which represents her new developing strength and creativity as she moves to a new level in her career.

She writes in her journal, "What sprouts are emerging in me now that need protection, care, and nourishment? I need to protect them from villainy and ignorance so my creativity can blossom. I need to refuse to accept authority from immoral sources.

"I need to question what I feel and know in my heart to be wrong, and to honor what I feel and know in my heart to be right.

"Where am I being the jokester? When am I casual and demeaning to my own developmental process? When and where do I ignore the fact that I need protection,

tenderness, love, wise teaching, and cherish-
ing?"

How would you answer Julie's journal
questions for your life situation? Can you
find the jokester in you who, with a casual
grin more oblivious than sadistic, extin-
guishes your creative spark? Do you prevent
your own warm fires from lighting your way
to a more expansive life? Did you believe
that when you moved into recovery you
would be free from obstacles that could stall
your ability to improve your life?

Your fantasies about what your recovery
would look like might have been as unrealistic as a child's fantasies about being an
adult. As you separate from your eating
disordered life, you will find yourself in situations that baffle you. However, in recovery
you recognize that your bafflement signifies
that you are in a realistic situation that your
eating disorder formerly blocked you from
acknowledging. You appreciate your need
for learning experiences that address these
situations or else your bafflement will cause
feelings of helplessness — an eating disorder
trigger.

In recovery you continually grow by caring for yourself. You tend those aspects of
yourself that need help. By living a self-
caring life, you tolerate your feelings of

helplessness because they do not define you. Instead of going to food for relief, hiding, or becoming fearful or shamed, you pause, gather yourself together, and rely on the knowledge that you can find ways to cope.

Like so many recovery exercises and activities in this book, many of your self-care practices have little to do with food or eating. You find that when you do the self-care exercises you feel confident, secure, and cared for. Your adult mind doesn't have to soothe a frightened and neglected internal child. You free your adult self to deal with your current situation.

For example, do you regularly clean and care for your body, clothes, bedding, home, and car? Do you make necessary repairs in an efficient and timely fashion?

Children can't do many of these things. When you tend to these self-care activities, you reassure the part of your psyche that is young and moving toward maturity. You earn your own trust and feel the security that comes with being in a clean, orderly, reliable, and safe environment.

How good are your eating habits? Do you eat sitting down; from a plate, not a container; three meals a day and two snacks, with appropriate amounts from all food groups?

Do you give yourself pleasurable eating experiences, like eating with a friend, eating in a park or garden, or listening to music while you eat? Do you have a mindful meal once a week?

Did you say no in a healthy and appropriate way to yourself or someone else and prevent a binge or a triggering activity that could lead to a binge? *Binge* here means bingeing on anything: eating, starving, exercise, shopping, drinking, anger, self-criticism, crying jag, TV, Internet, sex, drugs, or sleep deprivation. Give yourself credit for progress you are making and give yourself compassion for your attempts to do better.

Anything that alters or dims your consciousness can take you out of reality. Your recovery work is about staying here. Are you staying "here" more often and for longer periods of time? That's a goal to strive for and a win to celebrate.

Lack of sleep affects your consciousness, your emotions, your ability to think, your perceptions, your physical coordination, your memory, and your health in general. This information should chase us all to bed every night for at least eight hours. Yet we are a sleep-deprived nation.

Sleep deprivation serves a function if you

have an eating disorder. You know you use food to modulate your emotions and your awareness. You can use sleep deprivation the same way.

Do you delay going to sleep? Do you fall asleep on the couch while watching TV? Make an effort to give yourself a comfortable and cozy sleeping place and give yourself the eight hours you need to heal, nourish your mind and body, and be able to be present for the coming day. Reading children's bedtime stories to yourself in bed can bring you ease and help you drift off to a restful sleep.

In the space between wakefulness and sleeping is a time when you are particularly vulnerable to feelings. This can be a time to relax into creative associations that enrich your dreams and your psyche. It can also be a place where your increased vulnerability brings up anxiety.

Young children know this well. In the transition time between waking and sleeping the child needs lullabies and bedtime stories. She needs to be tucked in and kissed good night. She may need a glass of water or one more trip to the bathroom before she can settle down and drift into restful sleep.

You need that too. If you don't appreciate

that need, you will do what you can to avoid the transition time. If you force yourself to stay up beyond endurance, you will eventually skip over that vulnerable place and fall into a sleep that is more like passing out. Your sleep is brief and doesn't nourish you well.

Eight hours of sleep a night is your recovery goal. How many hours do you get now? Too much or too little will disrupt your consciousness and your health. Work toward increasing or decreasing your sleep to approach eight hours. The sleep you may need now is not a criterion for your sleep needs in the future. You need more sleep early in your recovery to make up for past deprivation and to help your body adjust to regular sleep nourishment and healing. You especially need adequate rest to restore your energy while you are going through the stress of moving on with your recovery work.

You may find that you sleep the way you eat, with periods of deprivation followed by bingeing. Some people try eating every other day. This stimulates more cravings and disrupts health and the ability to think. You may be doing this with your sleep behavior, depriving yourself of sleep during the week and giving yourself more sleep on the weekends. This disturbs your ability to think and modulate your emotions, and makes you more vulnerable to the seemingly quick fix of an eating disorder. Just as you need food in regular, reliable, and appropriate amounts every day to fuel your body, you need sleep in regular, reliable, and appropriate amounts every night, preferably in total darkness.

Give yourself credit for approaching adequate sleep. If you are not getting it, give yourself credit for striving toward it. Solutions to your current challenges may become clearer when you have a well rested and well nourished body and mind.

To develop satisfying and pleasurable sleep, experiment with the following practices:

Make your bed attractive with clean sheets, blankets, and pillows arranged nicely, close closet doors and bureau drawers, pick up clutter, make the room dark, don't have a mirror facing the bed, and place pen and paper and a glass of water at your bedside.

Once you are in bed, say out loud what is meaningful to you: a prayer, your affirmations, a supportive poem. When you wake, take a few minutes to lie in bed feeling whatever you are feeling. Then get your pen and paper and write down what you are feeling or your dreams or both. Care for yourself well on both sides of sleep.

Another check-in issue is laughter and play. How much and how often did you laugh and play this week? Reflect on who or what brought you pleasure and moments of joy. Are you learning to distinguish between being numb to pain and being happy? What will bring you more opportunity to laugh and play?

I can rely on the young children in my family, my terrier, Winston, and my improv class for play and uninhibited spontaneous laughter. Reach out and find your way to play.

Recovery includes many forms of personal enrichment. As you become more aware, you release your curiosity. Are you finding ways to honor your curiosity like taking a class; learning to use a computer, iPod, or Blackberry; or following a current event? Journal about ways you can pursue your curiosity.

If you have an eating disorder, you judge yourself harshly and treat yourself harshly when acting out your eating disorder. You are unaware that you are being harsh and cruel because your judgment and behavior are normal to you. You may be just as unaware with others.

Where have you been kind to yourself and other people? Kindness brings an end to self-punishment. Harshly criticizing your body, mind, or spirit is unkind.

Give yourself and other people kind and nourishing words, attention, and caring, especially when you or someone else feels low. Practice sentences like:

"I have confidence in you." "I'm sorry you are troubled. I have every confidence you will find your way through this challenge." "You have strength and wisdom you can rely on to see you through."

These statements, when you mean them, support and encourage. This is not people pleasing, speaking by rote, or sacrificing your own time and energy in an effort to rescue someone. You are not making yourself superior in knowledge or competence. You are sincerely directing your kindness toward a person to help them rally their own resources.

How are you doing with your affirmations? Have you created any of your own? Find or create affirmations that express your values and beliefs and what you want in your life, and how you want to behave.

You are on your recovery journey. You are being brave and determined as you move through your challenges to develop new ways to live in this world without your eating disorder. Real recovery doesn't happen fast, but it lasts.

Please remember this fundamental key to eating disorder recovery. You create the opportunity and conditions for your heart and soul, your body and mind, to heal and grow beyond your present limitations.

This check-in is designed to give you a sense of the territory you move through on your journey. You are not expected to simply check off every item with ease and a sense of completion. Many of these activities are new to you. Many of your eating disorder habits are so thoroughly ingrained that they seem normal.

Through the exercises in this book and the check-in process, you are chipping away at the structure, the habits, the mindset, and the beliefs that have locked you into the prison of your eating disorder.

You don't move through this rapidly. Even if you could, it wouldn't be a good idea. Moving through slowly gives you the experience of living a new and healthier way. Most importantly, it gives your entire being and emotional structure many gentle healing and growing experiences. You give yourself time to adjust to your new place in the world. You grow with each step so that you are capable of taking the next. Recognizing and honoring this part of your process is the ultimate kindness that will carry you through hard times and keep you healing and growing to freedom.

It's not uncommon in my psychotherapy practice for a client new in recovery to feel that she has become clumsy. She bumps into furniture or knocks her shoulder against the doorjamb as she leaves my office. She might stumble over the threshold.

She's not being clumsy. Her center of gravity is shifting. She is off balance because she is present emotionally and physically in a new way. She's not yet accustomed to her new normal, including the position of her body in space. She proceeds in her recovery work at a speed and level that matches her newly learned abilities to cope with change.

She needs to pause at each level as her mind, spirit, body, and sense of balance adjust. If she proceeds too fast, she will go beyond her ability to cope. That triggers feelings of fear and helplessness.

You can cope with a little fear and sense of helplessness as you move along on your recovery path. Too much, and you adjust back to your last level of recovery. You may need to journal more or bring back an exercise you thought you no longer needed.

Occasionally you will need to do this. Please don't criticize yourself when this happens. It's actually a time to celebrate because you went beyond your limits, recognized it, knew how to take care of yourself, and did. This is a great win in recovery.

Kindness, patience, and respect are key forces to further your development and progress. You build your ability to rely on your accomplishments and growing sense of how to care for yourself in the here and now.

DAILY EXERCISES

1. Follow your breath for ten minutes at least three times a day.
2. Read or recite your three affirmations twenty times at least three times a day.
3. Write about how you feel when you follow self-care practices. How do you feel when you enter you bedroom and the bed is made nicely; the bathroom is clean and organized; your favorite book and a glass of water are next to the bed?
4. Body scan at least three times a week.
5. Backtracking: Go back now and read your journal entries from when you

started working your way through this book. Journal on what you discover. If you discovered harshness, add a note of kindness to yourself on the page.

Chapter 12
Sex, Stalking, and Exploitation

"As long as you have certain desires about how it ought to be you can't see how it is."
— Ram Dass

The topic of sexuality is near the end of this book because, if you have been working the exercises in previous chapters, by now you are more equipped to look at this highly charged issue. I invite you to look at your sexual life through the lens of eating disorder recovery work. My intention is not to discuss sexual addiction, orgasmic dysfunction, or morality but rather to introduce a subject that is not discussed fully and openly as it relates to people with eating disorders.

What I know from my own personal experience and hear in my practice is this: The lived sexual experiences of women with eating disorders are acutely troublesome and remain largely unspoken in public discourse and in consulting rooms. They are characterized by many of the experiences described in the following list. Some of them may be familiar to you.

Please do your breathing exercise and look at this list without judgment. Follow the principles we looked at in Chapter 9, "Spiritual Depth."

Do any of these points reflect your experience now or in the past?

- Become aroused during foreplay but lose all sexual desire at penetration.
- Enjoy cuddling and simple foreplay but get frightened or numb when your partner's sexual energy becomes more intense.
- Become aroused by receiving or inflicting pain and humiliation.
- Have been harassed by a stalker.
- Have been a stalker in varying degrees in person or by phone.
- Have multiple affairs with married men, men in power, and men unavailable for committed relationship because of addictions or secrets.
- Have been faithful, loyal, and deferential to a man you thought was committed but who had a secret sexual life.

- Felt special while knowingly having sexual relations with a man who had many lovers yet you believed you were his favorite and that eventually you would be together.
- Have fled to bars looking for attention, flattery, and sex.
- Have repeatedly been disappointed when a brief encounter did not mean the beginning of a relationship.

If one or more of these experiences are part of your history or current life, looking at them can open emotionally loaded secrets. Please do not go into harsh judgment of yourself. Stay present, and look, perhaps for the first time, not at shoulds or should nots, but simply at what is.

If you have different items to add to this list, please do so. Anything about your sexual life that brings up shame, guilt, thrills, or disappointment belongs on this list.

These sexual experiences, seemingly intimate to you in the moment, often leave you lonely or feeling isolated or numb. You may feel close to the person you are sexually involved with but removed from others in your life because you must keep your liaison secret. Or you feel close to some people in your public life while your secret sexual activity is with strangers.

Marge, suffering from bulimia most of her life, only let herself be sexually involved with married men. She lived this way from ages twenty-seven to forty-five. She preferred that the men live out of town. Marge had a group of men who called her when they visited her city. She felt excited and special when she made plans with them on the phone. She had continual hopes for lavish weekends with them, and the first date or two satisfied her hopes as they stayed at expensive hotels and dined in fine restaurants. But that usually didn't last more than a few dates. She also believed that each man would be the fulfilling relationship in her life and would give her lush, romantic, satisfying sex, but her actual experiences felt sordid to her and rarely were sexually satisfying.

Marge did not understand why these men treated her as a free prostitute, yet, when one of the men developed a genuine caring for her, she was repulsed. For the most part, she kept her relationships with these men secret or left out the fact that they were married when she spoke of them.

Marge's pattern is not unusual. It's based on what could be described as adult insecurity because she is an adult in age, but her pattern is based on the goals and strivings of a young, immature psyche struggling to live an adult woman's life — the situation of any woman who suffers from an eating disorder. She feels unworthy, anxious, and incapable of being safe while receiving and giving.

Marge chose men who failed her. It never occurred to her that they were lying to her or that she was lying to them. She showed them she was available on their sporadic terms and had no idea that her wanting them to love her and treat her like a beloved princess would surprise them. Marge wanted love and a sense of security and believed these relationships fell far short of her wish because she was too unworthy or unlovable.

If this describes any part of your experiences, please breathe and do a simple body scan right now. Stay awake while you read what may bring this pattern into your life. Like Marge, do you respond immediately to possible partners who flood you with anticipation, phone you, and send you notes that give you respite from your loneliness and sense of worthlessness? If your answer is yes, you, like Marge, linger in private child-like fantasies of romantic splendor with these men. You deny your occasional glimpse of lies and sordidness, trying to protect and extend your fantasy. When the dream eventually crashes, you feel anger, disgust, great loss, a worthlessness, and a sense of failure and betrayal. You are a Cinderella with your coach destroyed, a menial dressed in rags again. Except in your story the prince does not come looking for you. You have to find another prince and live the story all over again.

Unlike Cinderella, you and Marge have little or no internal sense of worth or faith in yourself. (That's changing for you as you continue with your recovery work, and you can feel it.)

But the experience of losing your fantasy in this kind of relationship leaves you feeling bereft with nothing to sustain you. Although you feel grief and shame at where you find yourself, you look for a candidate who will bring back your sparkling fantasy as soon as possible.

This pattern becomes a psychological trail that can lead you to one-night stands, affairs while married, liaisons with employers, professors, and people of either gender who seem powerful and able to fulfill your immature yearnings.

In these experiences the man fills the gaps

in your psyche with false and temporary fantasies shored up by sexual attention and promises. When the relationship falls apart, you experience an inner collapse. You may fall yet again into your dark night of the soul.

The man's power to attract you does not necessarily have to be real power in this society. He may seem powerful to you because he is a rebel. He may reject education or a legal means of making a living, and he may use others to pay his way in life, living a life that seems glamorous to you.

You believe that his attention gives you the same superior status you believe he holds. In your fantasy, and perhaps his, you are above the rules of society.

The consequences of such a relationship vary according to your strength and self-esteem. On the low end of the continuum, the relationship parallels or becomes that of a pimp using his docile and obedient prostitute. The high end is when you grow from within, drop the fantasy yourself, and pull out of the connection as you build a healthy life for yourself. In recovery that's eventually what Marge did.

Isabel, suffering from compulsive overeating and binge eating, had a different but equally tragic pattern with men. She was attracted to Howard, a man who seemed to adore her and was inferior to her in every possible way. She felt safe with him because he grew to need her abilities in life and cherished her all the more for them. Howard was less educated than Isabel, made less money, lacked social graces, and failed to live up to his responsibilities at work or at home.

While she felt safe and often maternal toward him she also felt annoyed that she had to take charge in maintaining their home and their financial life plus guide him to be more competent in his job. She sometimes felt a sense of shame being with him. She was stunned and at a loss when he became abusive emotionally and physically. Yet she accepted his abuse because, when he called her "fat," he reinforced her own harsh judgments on herself and she felt lucky to have him in her life at all.

If Isabel's story seems familiar to you, then you know this kind of relationship can last many years. When Isabel began her recovery work, she was determined to maintain her fantasies about her wonderful life with Howard and how lucky she was to have him. By learning to be more present and capable of tolerating her feelings, she woke up. With her new awareness she discovered that Howard had been lying and cheating for years. In her recovery work, Isabel's immature psyche was maturing. Despite her pain and sorrow, she believed she deserved better.

When the relationship ended along with her fantasy she didn't collapse. Without realizing it and as part of her recovery, she had been building herself internally and creating powerful supports externally to hold her when her life fell apart. Her way of life fell apart, but she didn't.

She had some weeks when she felt, at times, like an abandoned child in a dangerous world, but these were short lived. The combination of her inner and outer support system held her much better than the fantasy of the relationship or her compulsive eating.

More sexual challenges exist for a woman with an eating disorder. It's not uncommon for new clients in my practice to have or to have had a stalker in their lives. Have you? A person, man or woman, stalks when they believe they love or have a right to possess another person. The stalker can't bear the anxiety they believe is caused by the other person's distance. I can't get into all the psychological combinations that create a stalker, but I do want to open up an exploration of how, when you live with an eating disorder, you may attract a stalker or become one. (See Reid Meloy's books listed in the references if you want to know more.)

Renee, a twenty-four-year-old bulimic, moved away from her home state to escape her controlling parents and start college. Her boyfriend, who had little money and no plans to go to college, joined her in Los Angeles. Renee and Jack shared a tiny apartment for a brief time, but Renee needed privacy to study. Jack moved out, but they saw each other every day. Renee grew more involved with her academics while Jack got involved in the Los Angeles drug scene. They spoke on the phone several times a day but rarely saw each other. Renee cried and wondered why he never had time for her and eventually after several months of not seeing him, told him, on the phone, that the relationship was over.

Jack stalked her. He called multiple times a day. He sent her ten or more long e-mails a day. In these messages he professed love and how much he needed her. He said his life and hers were not worth anything if they weren't together.

Renee needed this impaired man to accompany her to Los Angeles because she didn't have the internal cohesiveness to make the move alone. He went with her because he only felt whole with her. As long as they both remain impaired, they could fill each other with needed emotional support.

As Renee started to emerge as her own person, she no longer filled the gaps for Jack. He wanted the feeling of wholeness and power he only had with her. He didn't have to see her. Knowing she was available to him and contacting her by phone and e-mail was enough. But that limited contact was not enough for Renee, who wanted a full relationship. She had been using Jack the same way she used her eating disorder — to carry her through unbearable anxiety. When she took over even part of her own life, Jack couldn't accept the change and became a stalker.

Your protection against acquiring a stalker and against becoming one yourself is to become healthy, awake, and real to yourself. Then you are more able to see the reality of another person. You are not attracted to someone who "can't live without you," and you go to your recovery work if you begin to feel that way about someone else. With such awareness you can avoid or extricate yourself from predatory relationships.

Yet another sexual challenge involves secrets. If you have an active eating disorder and are in a romantic relationship where you keep secrets about your lover's life or even the existence of the relationship, you are in trouble. If you never doubt that he is being honest with you and that keeping his secrets proves your love and makes your relationship special, you are in trouble.

For example, if he has secrets you know about, he probably has secrets you don't know about. If you are in a relationship with a married man you believe loves you, you may not be able to imagine that he could be as unfaithful to you as he is to his wife.

You need to believe your fantasy about him to stay emotionally intact, and he needs a woman who believes that fantasy in order to keep his lifestyle intact. Again, these painful and sometimes dangerous relationships develop for the same reasons you developed an eating disorder. You can't establish self-caring and self-respecting boundaries; you can't tolerate your anxieties, and you are looking for what works to soothe you and make you feel powerful and loved.

Often these relationships leave you more wounded than you can admit to yourself or anyone else. You will most likely bury yourself more deeply in your eating disorder for escape, and that only increases your profound shame. Promising yourself that you will never have a relationship like this again or being eager to find another just like it with a happier ending is similar to your self-talk about your eating disorder. "I'll never throw up again." "I'll find the diet and exercise program that lets me eat what I want and be happy." Your true way out of these destructive patterns is to heal, and that involves helping a part of your psyche achieve maturity.

My granddaughters, Hannah and Delilah, continue to be teachers in my life. A game they and their friends play is "Prince and Princess." They dress up in filmy soft pink cloud dresses that twirl when they spin, and they dance. One part of the game is for Delilah to lie down and pretend she is a sleeping princess. Hannah pretends to be the prince. The prince approaches the sleeping princess (who is struggling not to smile), leans over her face, and plants a gentle kiss. This is "love's first kiss" that awakens the sleeping princess. With smiles of joy the princess leaps up, and they both dance happily at the wedding in the palace.

This naïve dream might be delightful play for young children, but it's a dangerous game for an adult woman. The eating-disordered woman often brings this level of naiveté to her relationships with men and finds herself suffering the sexual and emotional experiences described earlier.

As you age, you are confronted with the challenges of a complex world and are expected to cope as an adult woman. These challenges include relationship and sexual challenges. You may look like a woman and act like a woman because you are a woman, and you've studied the appropriate ways to behave, but you can be as naïve and vulnerable as a child in an adult sexual atmosphere.

Further, if you have an eating disorder, you strive to achieve a body that is beautiful by whatever your standards are. Those standards are usually unrealistic and based on childish beliefs. You strive for beauty because you genuinely believe it will bring you happiness, wanted attention, love, family, wealth, career, success, safety, security, or whatever it is that you want. You believe beauty will bring all the wonders and delights of love's first kiss.

The more your body is removed from that standard, the more miserable, angry, and despairing you become. You seek isolation because of what you consider to be your shameful appearance, or you flaunt your body in defiance of your shame.

A person who seems to offer you what the child in you believes to be real and possible touches your vulnerable yearnings. He can seem to be the prince, the powerful rescuer, the noble man, the wise or the knowledgeable or wealthy or devilishly clever one, the one who can shower you with all the treasures of your fantasies. In his eyes you are the most beautiful, desirable, and precious woman. He will make your life easy. He will elevate you above your everyday worries and surroundings. In his arms you are safe and home. This is the vision you see through the distorted perceptions of your eating disorder.

You have to do nothing except smile as he gives his all for you. If he doesn't, you are disappointed, sad, or angry. You might have a tantrum or pull away, isolate. Or you might use your eating disorder to help you see what isn't there. He may treat you badly and you make excuses for him, excuses you believe in order to keep your fairy tale alive.

In the classic fairy tales, the feminine is a heroine. She has tasks as well as the prince. Cinderella worked hard toward her own development and maturation — in the cinders, in the attic, in the fields, in the stable. She toiled in an environment of ashes, dirt, mice, and rats. Despite great loss and dark human emotions, she triumphed. She learned from her years of toil as she developed from child to competent woman — a woman capable of being not just a princess, but a queen of the land.

Children don't see the efforts that adults make to mature into people who can drive cars or ships or jets. It looks like magic to them. "When I grow up, I'm going to be a movie star," the child says with no sense at all of the effort involved in making that vision a reality. She imagines a life of beauty, ease, and delight where she wears pretty clothes and everyone loves her. Unfortunately, abbreviated versions of the fairy tales too often leave out the reality of hard work that goes into development and transformation.

What adds to the difficulty in exploring these issues is that in many ways you are a competent, intelligent, and realistic person. You have pockets of immaturity that your eating disorder lets you skip over, but what you feel and attract sexually gets confused between the raw needs of your underdeveloped psyche and your mature body.

When the child psyche in the woman's body attempts to cope in a sexual environment, it is painful. Like a child, you look to see and mimic what seems to be appropriate behavior without genuine maturity.

An eating disorder cuts you off from your genuine sexuality just as it cuts you off from your other feelings. You know about performing, faking, manipulating, and pretending. You know about cuddling and being frightened when cuddling changes to sexual intensity. You know about fear at penetration. You know about boredom and feeling nothing. You know about your need to please and your certainty that beauty will stimulate your partner. You try to catch hold of your partner's desire because you feel little of your own. Or you feel a great deal of passion and sexual intensity, but you have little awareness or interest in your partner's.

In many ways you are emotionally isolated. You crave affection. You are full of wishful fantasies. You experience loneliness and terrible emptiness and seek flooding sensations for relief. When you have an eating disorder you have no realistic way to cope with these feelings. You cross boundaries you don't see and move into experiences of exploitation and danger. Sadly, you can be exploited without realizing it because your way of life blocks your awareness. You can even be in danger while you believe your fantasies are coming true — at least for a while.

As you move into recovery, pockets of immaturity shrink. You notice things. You ask questions. You have opinions. You discover what you care about and develop the confidence and skills to pursue your authentic desires. You say no and honor your boundaries and your values.

If your sexual partner truly cares about you, they want you to be well and fulfilled. They will support your growth and be glad you are healing. They will gracefully or not so gracefully adjust to the changes in their life because of your changes. Part of your recovery work involves developing patience and compassion as people in your life make what may be difficult adjustments in order to relate to you as a more authentic and mature person.

For example, if an aspect of your relationship includes your husband or lover taking on major financial or social responsibilities because you are limited, that changes as you take on more, and he takes on less. If your partner depends on your eating-disordered oblivions and fantasies, what he may have hidden from you will be revealed. A new level of honesty will have to develop between the two of you. As you are more authentic, your relationship becomes more authentic.

This can be a relief or a challenge for the

people in your life. Some will object to your changes and not be able to adapt to your increased awareness and realistic presence. The issues of secrets and boundaries re-emerge here. As you give up your secrets because they are no longer necessary and as you create boundaries that allow your life to function in a healthy way, relationships that require secrecy and lies fall apart.

Exercises that address the troubling aspects of an eating-disordered woman's sexual life can be found in Appendix B. Many have little to do with sex.

Here are a few practices to consider bringing into your life:

1. Befriend your own body. Instead of punishing your body with criticism, poor nourishment, and grueling exercise, gift your body with nourishment, dance, yoga, or swimming.
2. Create nonsexual intimacy with friends by sharing passion about a cause you both believe in or by working together in an organization you both support.
3. Keep up your breathing exercises and body scans to increase your ability to remain present.
4. Discover pleasurable body sensa-

tions like walking, bathing, showering, enjoying the sun, and walking in the rain. (Georgia O'Keeffe painted a tree in a breeze with leaves swirling around the base of the trunk. When I saw that canvas, I remembered the delightful feeling of my lightweight skirt caught in a breeze and swirling around my lower body from hips to calves.)

5. Imagine a life in the future with a loving partner.

   Often this imagery includes a solid, loving marriage with children, family, friends, and pleasant relationships with people in your community. Write vivid and detailed descriptions of tiny moments with your fantasy potential husband such as the two of you getting the children ready for bed or breakfast on a weekday.

Over time you can use these developing stories of your womanly heart's desire as a way to look at others in your life. Does the married man, the secret lover, the charming seducer, the dependent clinger, the fun party guy fit into your dream?

You may not want a family. Perhaps your

children are grown. Your scenario may be that you and your lover travel together or run a business together or live a creative life where you paint or write or sculpt. Perhaps your imagery captures a quiet person who reads or spends time on the computer, is easygoing, and enjoys your flamboyance. Or perhaps he or she is the flamboyant social one who enjoys your quiet serenity. Fill in the details of the life you would like to live.

These projections can help you appreciate what you are sacrificing when you act out sexually. You develop motivation to heal and set your genuine boundaries so you can make better choices earlier.

If you have an eating disorder, you most likely know that while human sexuality is flagrantly advertised and exploited, demonized and idealized, your actual experience is rarely reflected back to you in ways that are realistic or help you understand yourself.

The media plays into your vulnerabilities. You can be just as harsh or even harsher on yourself than the impossible standards of beauty the media set for women. You believe you must have a certain look and be a certain weight or size before you are attractive, desirable, and lovable. Yet love has nothing to do with this standard or this judgment. Learning to accept yourself, love another, and allow yourself to be loved is a vital part of eating disorder recovery.

Healthy children teach us. Has a healthy, beautiful child with skin like silk worriedly pointed out to you a "boo-boo" you almost needed a magnifying glass to see? When Delilah did, I peered at the flaw. Her momentary dismay was untouched by shame. In a day her body was blemish-free again. She was confident all would be well and accepted quite naturally that, indeed, all was well.

Perhaps you maintain your childhood belief that body perfection is your normal condition. Do you believe that any disturbance in that picture is a worrisome catastrophe that warrants your being an outcast or your need to hide in disguising clothes? If this is you, then, like a child, you cannot yet relate to the human experience of physical changes brought by aging, illness, weight gain, weight loss, accidental disfigurements, and battle scars. Somewhere in your mixed perceptions of fantasy and reality is the child's expectation of body perfection and your belief that perfect beauty is essential in order to be loved.

Here's a suggestion I give my clients who are caught in their false beliefs about body appearance and love. I tell them to go to shops, malls, and parks and look for men and women who do not qualify as beautiful by your standards yet are holding hands or kissing. See them pushing strollers with smiling babies, or laughing and playing together, or sharing a tender moment.

People watching at the airport, train station, or bus station is good for this. Greetings and farewells bring up visible emotion in people of all sizes, ages, and shapes. Let these scenes from everyday reality — not reality TV — be your teacher.

My clients return from doing this exercise saying, "How can this be? I saw a fat woman looking happy and comfortable with a nice man and children," or "I can't understand how that old woman I saw in the restaurant could laugh like a sexy young girl with a handsome man who held her hand. I think he was her husband." These visions from real life shake up your beliefs about who is allowed to be loved and free you to accept yourself as you are.

With your budding awareness and growing sense of adulthood, determine if a potential liaison is a good real man or a childhood fantasy fulfillment or a predator. This is where your self-acceptance, your breathing exercises, and practices in being present will equip you to discern what or who is truly good for you. Attend to the person who attracts you in the same mindful way you've been doing your exercises. Drop your desires or wishes. Stay in the present and be aware as the person before you reveals himself.

Stay real. Don't let your insecurities be soothed and erased if he elevates you to a high status. Be wary if he expects you to appreciate how terrible other women were in his life, how they deserved what they got, how noble or misunderstood he is, or how he suffered with loneliness and pain because of the way others treated him. Stay real, or you will be the woman he's talking about to his next target.

When you are real, self-accepting, and respectful of boundaries, you recognize a man who is present, respectful, and genuinely interested in discovering who you are. With no secrets to keep, you explore openly the possibilities of a satisfying and fulfilling relationship.

The exercises and activities in Appendix B will inspire you, nourish you, and support you as you care for the developing young part of your psyche. By following them you allow your inner parts to catch up with each other and integrate. The naïve parts of yourself mature as you grow more aware and competent.

This kind of development and freedom allows you to connect, join, love, and share your life with others who are healthy and free. Yes, such people exist, but you can't see them or have access to them when you are in the grip of your eating disorder behaviors and mindset. As you become more kind, compassionate, and respectful of yourself, you are more able to see and receive kindness, love, and respect from others. You won't have to accept poor substitutes and fantasies to find moments of false security. The more real you become, the more wonderfully real your life can be.

You are developing safety and prevention experiences that help you recognize an incipient stalker or an exploiter. When you are more real to yourself, you are more able to see the reality of the person you are with. With that knowledge you are able to extricate yourself and protect yourself from predators.

DAILY EXERCISES

1. Follow your breath for ten minutes at least three times a day.
2. Read or recite your three affirmations

twenty times at least three times a day.

3. Backtrack a current or past sexual liaison that brought you pain, shame, guilt, or fear. Begin with the first clear moment you remember. Notice what was happening in that relationship a day and a week earlier, how you met, how you felt when you met and what was going on in your life. See if you can discover what fantasies you wanted that person to fulfill.

4. Write about the kinds of sexual liaisons that are dangerous for you. Ask yourself, "How can I know when I am in physical or emotional danger? How can I recognize the true cost of being in these relationships, whether they are one-night stands or long term?" Also write about the heroes in your childhood dreams/fantasies. See any parallels?

CHAPTER 13
FAMILY

"The last of the human freedoms is to choose one's attitude in any given set of circumstances."
— Victor Frankl

Expectations and assumptions, fantasies and reality, love and anger, disappointment and hope, all crash together when you consider your family. In or out of your eating disorder, family visits, communications, and memories may be your most challenging experiences. The family you grew up with is made up of the people who were part of your environment while you were developing your eating disorder. You may have spent years relating to them with an eating disorder as part of your coping mechanism.

If you are married with a family of your own now, you have been living a life with them, too, as a woman with an eating disorder. In ways you and they know and don't know, everyone has adapted, for good or ill, to the psychological dynamics created by the eating disorder.

This doesn't mean you are at fault. You were or still are living in an environment where you need to develop or maintain an eating disorder to survive. That doesn't mean your family is to blame. It means the conditions necessary for your eating disorder to develop were and may still be present. Often the family doesn't change. In recovery, you take the lead. You change because you are going for freedom, health, and a better life. Nowhere will your commitment be more tested than with your family.

Part of recovery is tolerating complex feelings. When you are with your family and not bingeing or purging or starving, you can feel an inner roar when anger, guilt, fear, and resentment mix with love, duty, respect, and hope. Especially in early recovery, you expect the members of your family to understand your challenges and be supportive. This is complicated.

Sometimes you want them to give you room to practice your eating disorder, and sometimes you want them to give you room to be the healthy, more outspoken, free woman you're becoming. You and they can become frustrated and bewildered. Emotions can run high. You need to be able to sort the challenges inherent in your family relationships.

Your mother and father, your brothers and sisters, without knowledge or intention, sorely test you by their predictable habits. You are learning to use your new-found strengths and resources to help you care for yourself. You work to withstand the force of eating disorder triggers, and they abound when you are with your family.

You need to be kind to yourself, forgiving of yourself, and at the same time, search out and discover what triggers your eating disorder.

Your family does not know or understand your struggles or the specific nature of your healing work. Your new ways jar their expectations. They may feel hurt or angry by your unexpected behavior. Even if everyone in the home of your childhood behaved with great respect toward you, as a healthy adult woman simply being with them in old familiar settings can trigger you.

I remember in early recovery opening my parents' refrigerator. I gasped, shut the door quickly and took a walk around the house breathing to regain my equilibrium. The refrigerator was filled with their favorite foods and snacks: bags of Hershey Kisses, cups of chocolate pudding, bowls of leftover spaghetti, and large wedges of Camembert cheese. It was a sumptuous buffet of my binge and trigger foods — the foods I grew up with, loaded with emotional associations.

If I had encountered these foods in the course of ordinary living with my eating disorder, they might have triggered me into a full-blown binge/purge episode. As I recovered, my binge foods had less influence over my emotional state. That day, however, seeing all of my binge foods as I experienced them as a child, stored in the same way, some in the same dishes, felt like a full scale attack on my ability to remain stable.

In the family environment, you are more vulnerable to your eating disorder. You are tested by being in familiar rooms, seeing familiar faces, and hearing familiar stories and ways of speaking. Your challenge, as always, is to remain present and not act out. You need to appreciate and understand your experiences with your family without blaming them or blaming yourself when inevitable conflict occurs.

Many of your trigger foods are probably the same foods your family still eats. Adding to your stress is your mother's or aunt's or grandmother's voice saying, "It's your favorite. I made it for you. Have some." If you seem reluctant to accept, your stress increases when your father or uncle or grandfather says, "Oh, go ahead. She worked so hard to make this for you. A little won't hurt."

You feel pressure. You feel awkward, guilty, anxious, and angry at the people pushing you to eat. You also feel an inclination to sink back into your adolescent life and behave as they expect you to behave. Your anger increases because you believe they are creating a situation that is undermining your recovery. Some of your anger comes from your attempt to fight off your own temptation. You are primed to cry, blow up in rage, or attack. You need your recovery strength to breathe and stay present.

Draw on the benefits of your recovery work to negotiate family gatherings more peaceably. It can be done. You have options and choices.

First, don't visit your family when you are raw and vulnerable. Before you spend time with them, prepare. If your family is nearby, keep visits short when you are in early recovery. Before long or short visits, go through the following exercise in advance.

Look at your expectations: are they reasonable or wishful thinking? Perhaps your expectations bring up fear and anticipation of conflict. Keep breathing. Bring yourself to the present.

You don't know where your specific triggers will emerge when you are with your family. Use your adult resources to help you when emotions escalate and eating disorder urges are strong.

To do this establish your route to equilibrium in advance. For example, make arrangements to call your therapist or a friend or another supportive person in your life at specific times while you are with your family. Knowing you have that appointment will give you structure and remind you that you are visiting, not going back in time to live with them as the child you were. Speaking to your support person and hearing her voice is stabilizing when you feel anxious or highly emotional.

Journal when you are with your family about what you see and experience that is pleasant and unpleasant. Remind yourself that you can be present for both. You can also repeat your affirmations as you look at objects in your family's home that are emotionally charged for you.

By doing this you are building a bridge between your adult recovering self and the child you were. Assume that all the quirks, idiosyncrasies, assumptions, expectations, rituals, and patterns in your family are the same. This is how they lead their lives with you or without you. Does your father eat heavy foods after dinner while watching television? Does he drink too much? Does your mother clean the kitchen to a sparkling perfection? Does she relax by taking a tranquilizer or two? Does one criticize the other? Do they criticize others? Do they have their own ways of teasing or arguing or confounding one another that drove you crazy when you lived with them? Did you ever tell them how their behaviors affected you? Did you even know?

You can elaborate on your self-care plans in case their normal family routines and behaviors trigger you. Identify realistic options. For example, you might quietly read, make a phone call, take a walk alone or with the dog, play outside with a child, take a nap, or offer to help someone with a chore. You don't run, fight, or act out. You do the exercises and activities that support and ground you. You align yourself differently within the family system by relying on self-caring actions you choose for yourself. You don't get pulled in.

Your top priority and ultimate goal is to be healthy and whole. You want to be your own woman, free from the clutches, protection, and imprisonment of your eating disorder. To achieve this, you have to heal and grow from within. You know this now.

But it's easy to forget when you are with family!

To help you stay on your recovery path with your family, see Appendix B for Chapter 13 exercises. Create new affirmations that are specific to triggering situations with your family.

Your challenge is to be in recovery in this world as it is. That includes being with your family as they are, but it doesn't mean that you adapt to situations that threaten your recovery.

Your fundamental standard, when visiting your family, is to be kind, gracious, and caring while remaining firm in your ability to say no to requests or assumptions contrary to your health and well-being.

In your family environment, eat on a regular basis. Let your family know in advance that you are making eating choices based on your health needs today. They can serve whatever foods they wish. You will work your way around what they have or go shopping to stock food that is right for you. You might offer to cook them a dinner, or one dish to add to their menu, based on your new way of eating.

When the pressure comes, as it inevitably does, for you to eat what you cannot or should not, you need to be firm when you decline. Let them feel what they may feel. You can quietly do your breathing exercise at a dining room table, in a car, or at a restaurant while they absorb your "no."

You no longer take on responsibilities that are not yours. You feel your feelings. You stay present for what is, including people having their feelings. You remain present while the people around you are surprised, disappointed, mocking, angry, befuddled, or sad. This kind of situation comes up often in early recovery and is a tough test for you. You learn to be graceful in such situations. Saying your truth, like "No, thank you," breathing, gathering your inner resources, and being quiet supports your recovery more than you may yet appreciate.

Because you are learning to tolerate your feelings without engaging in your eating disorder behaviors, you are also learning that feelings can be tolerated. You know that feeling won't hurt you or kill you. This growing knowledge helps you be still while the people in your family feel their own feelings. You don't have to defer, postpone, or eliminate your self-respect, your recovery needs, your self-esteem, or your deeply held values. Your recovery is upsetting their status quo. Give them a chance to learn to be with you as you are.

If pressure continues for you to behave and respond as you did in the past with your eating disorder to get you through, repeat, "No, thank you," continue to breathe, and stay in your recovery mode. Your family may not be accustomed to your creating boundaries. The people in your life, whoever they are, will be meeting you as you are now. They are meeting a woman in recovery who is considerate of other people, present in the moment, self-caring, and who sets necessary boundaries to honor her recovery work.

Being assured of privacy for sleeping, journaling, and meditating is important so you can rest with what you are feeling and thinking, especially during long visits. This may mean that others have to wait or adjust their plans. How they respond is up to them. You are not responsible for their assumptions. Of course, you let them know your needs in advance so they have an opportunity to make realistic plans.

As you have more time in your recovery, you will grow more at ease with your family. In the early stages, you need support and tools for maintaining your recovery and your relationships. Before spending time with your family, prepare by making arrangements and reinforcing your recovery commitments. Continue your recovery practices during your visit.

However, it's possible to think so much about your recovery work and the triggering forces within your family that you forget your family's lovable and admirable qualities.

As part of your preparation for being with them, answer these questions. What do you enjoy about your family? What do you admire about each family member? What valuable lessons or good habits did they teach you?

Remember good times — playing checkers, going through old jewelry with Mother and listening to stories, gardening with your parents, arranging and rearranging home decorations, making the bed together, neighborhood walks, doing crossword puzzles or playing board games, listening to music, dancing, singing, or talking about work or school or theater or sports.

Whenever you feel a lull or tension or awkwardness building, see if you can change the mood by suggesting an activity you know they enjoy and have enjoyed with you in the past. Be sure your suggestion is not in conflict with your recovery program.

To maintain your recovery progress, stay aware of what you need for your well-being. Sometimes what you need is love. As you appreciate now, a person with an eating disorder blocks intolerable feelings. She does what she can to avoid feeling vulnerable. In order to be aware and feel love coming to you from another person, you must be open to feeling and allow yourself to naturally respond. This is making yourself vulnerable.

Some people suffering from eating disorders are not loved, but many people with eating disorders are. The eating disorder defense prevents them from feeling or taking it in. They need proofs via gifts or obedience or attention, none of which is satisfying or reassuring. Is it possible that love is around you, but you can't recognize it or let it in? Part of your self-care is learning not to demand or expect love, but to create internal channels where existing love can flow to and from you. Your recovery involves learning to recognize and welcome love.

When you are with family, they are probably expecting the usual, whatever that may be. You have been doing work on yourself to be stronger, healthier, and more intact as a person. In blatant and subtle ways, you are changing. If they are not doing internal work on themselves, they will expect your time with them to be as it was in the past when you were deep in your eating disorder.

They will make assumptions they've always made and which you have accepted in the normal course of being with them. You are now working your way toward a "new normal," and that will bring up surprises, sometimes unpleasant ones.

Marianne, new in recovery, was single. Her cousins were married. On family visits, they had the guest room while she slept on the living room couch. She didn't sleep well, felt anxious, and wound up at night bingeing and trying to throw up quietly. The family was shocked and criticized her when she announced that she needed her own room during visits. Giving her a private room disrupted the usual arrangements.

She cried, felt guilty, undeserving, not worth being cared for or treated as an adult, but she expressed all that on the phone with her therapist, not with them.

With them, although she did have some tears, she let them know she loved them, she wanted to be with them, but for her own self-care and to honor her recovery work, she needed her own room. If that couldn't be arranged, she would be sorry not to join them on this visit, but her recovery had to come first. The disgruntled yet loving family found a way to accommodate her.

She was more at ease during that visit. She learned she could assert herself for her own genuine self-care needs. While her family was confused, upset that the routine was disrupted, and didn't understand the significance of what she asked, no one collapsed. No one got hurt. She learned she could make herself safe and comfortable without relying on her eating disorder. She now had evidence that she was more intact and sturdy than she had been. She now knew that others could survive her growing health. At this point there was no going back. She entered her "new normal."

When you sense you are near a triggering situation with your family, stay present and ask yourself, "What do I need for my psychological, physical, intellectual, or spiritual nourishment?" Keep in mind what you've learned from your recovery practices. You are not asking what others can do for you or how they can change for you.

Your answers to what you need will determine the boundaries you establish with your family that allow you to care for the whole adult woman you are. You are discovering who that woman is. Your family will learn who you truly are as you introduce yourself as that woman to them. To grow into your whole identity with no eating disorder to smooth away your anxieties, you will need to use your increasing strength and maturity to care for yourself. As you do this, your family will notice the change and learn the change is permanent. You are not going back to the old ways that triggered your eating disorder. You are becoming a free woman.

DAILY EXERCISES

1. Follow your breath for ten minutes at least three times a day.
2. Read or recite your three affirmations twenty times at least three times a day.
3. Write as many ways as you can think of to say "Thank you" for the gifts and helpful teachings you've received from your family. They hurt you and helped you. They took away and they gave. Explore how your family contributed to any of the strengths, interests, skills, insights, and competence you have.
4. Forward Track. This is a new exer-

cise. Go back to a time in your child-hood. See the child you were. Gently bring her through the years to your adult life. Show her how you live now. Then show her a future where you will take care of her, protect her, cher-ish her, and teach her how to live in the present moment. Tell her that you welcome her ability to be playful, creative, and curious. Tell her you will be happy to have her poke you when you are too serious and forget to laugh and dance.

Chapter 14
Triggers as Teachers: Staying on Your Recovery Path

"Commitment is what you stand on to breathe, attend to your body sensations, and courageously make your mindful moves."
— Joanna Poppink

You hit bumps on your recovery path and stumble or fall, as anyone does on a path into the unknown. Bumps in recovery are triggers that can release an emotional experience that sets off your eating disorder behavior. In recovery you change the effect a trigger has upon you. Moreover, you can use your triggers as teachers to help you progress on your recovery path.

Triggers come in many forms, often not frightening in and of themselves. Learning to recognize triggers that are unique to you is crucial for sustaining recovery. You plan how you will care for yourself when they appear. You need stamina to actuate your plan instead of your eating disorder.

Your eating disorder trigger stirs anxiety and evokes the feeling that you have no way to care for yourself. You do not need your eating disorder behaviors when you have a backlog of recovery work that equips you to be present for what threatens you.

To identify your triggers, go through your journal and spot situations that set off your eating disorder behaviors.

Separations of any kind are reliable, recurrent, and unavoidable triggers. Anything that involves change involves separation as you move from one condition to another. Even opportunities to advance your life or fulfill your dreams can be major triggers.

When you experience a trigger, your anxiety skips over your mind and sends an SOS to your body. You act out your eating disorder. When your eating or starving or excessive exercising subdues your anxiety, your body sends signals to your frightened self that all is well. You can stop or start eating or get off the treadmill.

In this situation and before your recovery work, "all is well" means that you've gotten to the other side of your triggering episode. You may be in a drugged state from eating. You may be passed out on the floor from vomiting. You may feel calm and able to wear your social façade in public with no blatant signs of your acting out. You may feel proud and relieved. You may feel isolated but special because your acquaintances and intimates don't know what you've been through. Your mind is more peaceful, and you have no reason to act out to protect yourself. You consider yourself safe.

A situation or a memory or an association that pierces your false façade and threatens your undeveloped psyche is a trigger to go into self-protective mode. Before recovery your protection is your eating disorder.

In eating disorder recovery, you work to heal, strengthen, and develop your psyche so you can deal with what life offers without needing to depend on your body to obliterate your mind and emotions. You explore your emotions to discover what frightened you and use your established recovery resources to care for yourself. Your body becomes a real player in your perceptions and decision making as you integrate the emotional, intellectual, spiritual, and physical aspects of yourself.

When you tolerate your anxiety, you discover that your body has its own rhythms. It will tell you when you need sleep or nourishment and how much plus alert you to real danger once you understand and listen to how your body speaks to you.

To remain in recovery, you need your body, mind, and spirit in harmony with one another. When one flounders, your eating disorder will rise to the occasion, like an understudy waiting for the star to fall ill.

Regardless of the specific nature of your eating disorder, you have used countless diets, exercise programs, and perhaps surgeries to trick your body into not needing or wanting what it needs. Recovery means your mind, emotions, and spirit cooperate with your body and distribute responsibilities in a fair and reasonable way. This gives you an opportunity to discover what your new found integration can accomplish.

When you want to dip into your eating disorder to soothe yourself, you have experienced a mild trigger, like a ripple in the sea. Your breathing and PAM exercises can get you through without acting out. You can journal later to find some insight into what that trigger means to you and where it gets its power.

When you feel a powerful urge to dive into your eating disorder to save yourself, you experienced a major trigger, like a rogue wave unexpectedly rising with the power to carry you out to sea. To weather this assault on your equilibrium, marshal the strength and awareness you've developed by using the following exercise.

Sit erect, perhaps with a pillow behind your back, on a sturdy chair with your legs uncrossed and your feet on the floor. Do a three-minute mindful breathing exercise. Pick up one foot, and place it to the side. Your foot has to be in one place before you can move it to another place. Make slight body adjustments so you feel in balance and secure. You are safe. Nothing major has changed, but separation has occurred. Your foot was in one place and now is in another. The place where it was is vacant. Your foot is adjusting to being in a new place, and your other foot is adjusting to a new space around it.

You are allowing your body to teach your psyche that you are present, you can move, you can tolerate shifts. Your body is teaching your psyche what is real.

Now stand and do three minutes of your breathing exercise. Then lift one foot and take a step. You are leaving one place for another place. Lift your other foot to take another step. You move beyond the place where your other foot stood. Now you have completely left the spot where you originally were standing.

Although this seems like simplicity itself,

you may find this exercise requires massive concentration and determination when you are confronting a major trigger. You remain emotionally present and aware while your body safely moves through simple states of separation. You bring your adult wisdom and strength to your frightened child psyche.

By doing this you increase your awareness of yourself, your body, and your existence in time and space. You are not dissolving or disappearing. Your body is showing you, through physical action that cannot be denied, that you are present and functioning. You didn't act out your eating disorder, and both your terror and cravings urge passed. You'll remember this.

In this exercise you also are learning the difference between the escape of distraction and the presence of mindfulness. You can walk at any speed when you are distracted from your body and receive no benefits. Mindful walking gives you physical evidence that you can survive separation, one step at a time. You learn that when you separate from one place you are immediately in place somewhere else. You are always "here."

Forcing yourself to be present when you are over taxed and under more pressure than you can bear can cause you to collapse into your eating disorder. You can stay present by expanding your present. Then you can refresh yourself and return to your challenge while remaining aware of your experience. This will develop as your awareness expands through your mindfulness practices.

For example, while driving past a park you see a traffic light ahead. You are "here" at the park. The traffic light is "there," a place you will never be because you are always here. But if "here" is the entire stretch of road, your "here" includes the park and the traffic light. You can extend your "here" to include the entire town or community or state. An advanced mindfulness practitioner can spread her awareness of "here" to include the entire planet and beyond.

With this expanded awareness you dissolve or deactivate triggers so they are smaller and have far less impact on you. In your expanded present you can give yourself ease with a book, a walk, silence, or play while still being present for your trigger. Your trigger weakens considerably as you experience the reality of who you are in the here and now.

Recovery brings you here. The more you can bear to be here, the less you are agonizingly nowhere and the less you need oblivion. You understand this now, but it's easy to forget when a trigger hits home.

Triggers are hooks that summon emotional experiences of other times when you were frightened, harmed, and helpless. When you succumb to a trigger, you feel a sense of guilt, shame, and failure as you add another layer of fear, punishment, and helplessness to your original experience. In this way the power of triggers intensifies over time.

A continuing honest and kind appraisal of yourself is necessary to protect yourself and weather your triggering experiences. You need to know your weaknesses so you can care for yourself well. This requires giving up feelings of entitlement or of being special and superior. You've developed those feelings as a result of the façade you built to hide your insecurities and your eating disorder. You come to believe the lie you present to others until a trigger destroys both your façade and your belief in the lies you've told yourself.

Self-honesty allows you to examine your genuine situation. Every exercise and activity in this book is designed to help you do that. The practices you've done and the practices on standby for when you are ready to use them are designed to help you develop the vision and stamina to be real to yourself.

Separation in the context of triggers covers a multitude of experiences and, for that reason, can take you by surprise. You may not make the connection between your desire to act out and the triggering event.

A store shuts down. A tree is cut down. A neighbor you barely knew moves away. This loss in your environment may disturb your precarious sense of security and reliance on an unchanging familiar. Divorce; a child leaving home for college, a job, or to be married; or a friend leaving town may leave you bereft with no way to adjust. Minor separations, like guests leaving your home after a social gathering, can trigger you because their leaving sparks your emotional memories of major separations.

Triggers can emerge out of your own imagination. You may awaken after a nightmare with overwhelming anxiety that drives you under the covers and later sends you groping for binge food or a full binge/purge episode.

Trigger foods are binge foods and vice versa. A binge food is your exit route from here. You see them, you taste them, and you know you can dive into them and be gone. They are like little spaceships you can ride fast out of this world. Some examples are pancakes, ice cream, frozen yogurt, pasta (that was one of mine), chocolate mints, and popcorn. Seeing them can trigger a binge. Learn to recognize yours.

The power of a trigger fades as you develop effective ways of dealing with what causes your stress. Frozen yogurt won't look like a rescue spacecraft when you stop to ask why.

People can be triggers when they challenge you to be present and real, such as someone reviewing your qualifications, face to face, for a job or school admission, or in social situations where someone is deciding whether you qualify as a friend or a date or a second date. Old entrenched and negative beliefs about yourself rise up in triggering moments.

The best preparation for coping well with triggers is to be healthy, self-caring, and emotionally sturdy so they don't send you into precarious states. Until that day arrives — and it will arrive if you stay on your recovery path — you can prepare yourself with the knowledge, skills, support, and reality checks you need. Continue your journaling, breathing, affirmation, and self-care practices.

Attending or having access to support

groups, your psychotherapist, an exercise program (preferably in a group, like a yoga class), social activities, and scheduled adult classes provide you with a nourishing and stabilizing routine. If a triggering event occurs, it does not take up the whole of your existence. You have people and activities in place to fill the void. You may feel as if you are about to fall into that void, but you show up where people expect you. By showing up, you learn that your world did not fall apart. You put one foot in front of the other and be present, defying your fears. If you don't show up, someone will call to find out where and how you are. You are not forgotten. Others hold you in their minds and hearts.

Living life without an eating disorder means living at a deeper level where you perceive more in the world, in other people, and in yourself. When you depend on your eating disorder, you want your resources readily available: binge foods, privacy to act out, adequate bathrooms and plumbing for purging, a treadmill at home and/or easy access to a gym. When you are in recovery, you want your resources readily available to maintain your recovery.

What would help you at 3:00 a.m. when you are anxious and feeling an urge to binge? What would help you when someone offers you candy at work? What would help you when someone comments on your body and you cringe with shame and want to act out?

First, make a list of situations that trigger you. Then think of what would help you ride through those experiences in a self-caring way. Remember to start with your breathing exercise. Here are several ways to give yourself recovery resources:

- Call a friend.
- Read or recite a supportive poem.
- Pull out and read affirmations you carry in your pocket.
- Excuse yourself and walk away.
- Phone exit strategies: "I'll call you back when I can," or "No, thank you," then hang up. "No, thank you," can help you out of many triggering situations.

In recovery you've developed strength and stability. Say no to people and activities that are bad for you. You are not pulled into negative activities because you are silent or give a weak yes that you don't mean. You follow a reasonable and healthy diet plan where you eat nourishing food at least every four hours without going to excess, without rushing to a scale, and without throwing up. You are not afraid of snacks and can have a cookie without it leading to ten more. You spend time alone without feeling isolated and depressed.

You listen to your mother or father or brother or sister say things that used to trigger you and are okay. You might be calm or angry and frustrated, but you don't attack or collapse. You don't allow the painful experience to last more than a few moments. You know how to extricate yourself from threatening scenarios, and you don't act out your eating disorder.

When an unexpected trigger rocks you like an earthquake, you can be the response to your own 911 call and use the recovery resources you've put in place. It's like having a fire extinguisher at the ready so a spark doesn't burn down your house. Maybe you haven't been following your exercises or using your resources for a while. Maybe you never tried some exercises because they seemed silly or irrelevant.

You can leave your resources, but they remain present. You can return to them. Your recovery resources are yours forever. You're only required to do one thing, and that is to remember them.

You are now committed to your recovery. That means that when everything falls apart and there is no one or nothing that seems stable or reliable, you still have your commitment. Commitment is there for when nothing else is. Commitment is what you stand on to breathe, attend to your body sensations, and courageously make your mindful moves.

You can reach for poetry, children's stories, exercise (swim, walk, jump rope, trampoline), runes, or your old journals. You can write out your fantasies, wishes, nightmares, day-mares, and dreams. You can call a "safe" friend, not like people from the old days who would gladly binge or drink or have sex with you while you are in this vulnerable state. As your equilibrium returns, though still shaky, you write what was going on in your life and in your fantasies in the hours and days leading up to your episode.

I don't like to use the word "relapse." Relapse means that you have gone back to where you were. You haven't. You can't. You are where you are now. Many events that used to trigger you do not trigger you anymore, because you've been doing your homework. You've become appreciative and respectful of yourself, more capable of meeting challenges.

A trigger signals that you have a vulnerable spot not yet resolved. It's like an arrow pointing to the buried treasure on the map. The treasure was buried so deeply that you didn't have a clue it was there. Your episode lets you know the location of a vulnerability that needs attention.

In this way your triggers become your teachers. They draw attention to where you need to grow, develop, and learn more self-care tools. As you give them mindful attention and use your developing resources, they guide you to new information about yourself and your life. They encourage you, by rattling your status quo, to explore beyond your current limits to learn and grow. As you meet your growth challenges, you grow more confident that you can meet your fears and still live well. This life in recovery is not a false promise or a fantasy. You are becoming a healthy and free adult woman capable of caring for herself, who is loving and loved.

DAILY EXERCISES

1. Do ten minutes of mindful breathing three times a day.
2. Read or recite three affirmations

twenty times morning, noon, and night. See Appendix A, "Affirmations."
3. Journal on the chapter titles of this book.
4. Backtrack from working through this book.
5. Forward Track: Imagine a wonderful life for yourself in solid recovery when you are decades older than you are. Describe one day in detail. Then backtrack from that day to learn what you did to create that future life.

APPENDIX A
AFFIRMATIONS

1. I happily nourish my body and am satisfied with moderate meals daily.
2. I welcome all my feelings knowing they guide me to my true self.
3. I deserve love and respect as I am.
4. I enjoy excellent health.
5. I have abundant energy.
6. I enjoy the colors, smells, and feel of life around me.
7. I am confident in the workings of my mind.
8. I am trustworthy. I can rely on me.
9. I say yes only when I mean it.
10. I say no when I feel it and mean it.
11. I am efficient and creative in my work.
12. I have ample time to relax and enjoy life.
13. I am lovable.
14. I delight in learning. I take classes and read books on subjects new to me.
15. I invite friends to join me in simple

pleasures.

18. I honor my mind, my body, and my spirit every day.
19. I give myself respect and encouragement as I move on my healing path.
20. I stand up for what I believe.
21. I am honest.
22. I care for myself.
23. I forgive myself for all the hurts I have inflicted on myself.
24. I am intelligent.
25. People are glad to support me.
26. I am getting better and better in every way.
27. I am a good age to be.
28. I tolerate my feelings.
29. I act or I do not act in the best interest of all concerned.
30. I am sexy and strong.
31. My courage unifies me.
32. I know what I know.
33. I shift from a limiting mental state to a limitless mental state easily and consistently.
34. I live in an endless sequence of now moments.
35. I know when to let go and move on.
36. I explore where my creativity and bliss lead me.
37. I use anxiety to create.

38. I get adequate rest, exercise, and nour-
    ishment.
39. People are happy to accept me.
40. I succeed where I put my efforts.
41. Timely right action and correct conduct
    are my true protection.
42. I am beautiful.
43. I complete my tasks.
44. I attract healthy, honest people into my
    life.
45. I interact with new people.
46. I am glad to be alive.
47. I exult in the success of others.
48. I keep my word to others.
49. I am courteous to myself and others.
50. People in my life are present for our
    mutual learning.
51. I expect the best.
52. I contribute to the happiness of others.
53. I follow through.
54. I ask for what I want.
55. I honor my schedule and responsibili-
    ties.
56. I honor my integrity and the integrity of
    others.
57. I am getting better and better in every
    way.
58. I'm a good friend.
59. I accept others as they are.
60. I treat humiliation as a teacher that

helps me get my priorities straight.

61. I create opportunities.

62. I turn knowledge into positive action.

63. I manage large and small sums of money well.

64. I am paid very well in money and respect.

65. I am prosperous and happy.

66. I am glad to be publicly accountable.

67. I let others help.

68. I am desirable.

69. I make amends promptly with a steady presence.

70. I deserve success.

71. I attend to practical, concrete matters.

72. I tolerate others' anger and disappointment and remain true to myself.

73. People are glad to be with me.

74. I am willing to succeed.

75. I breathe, enjoy, am honest, listen, learn, ask for what I want, and follow my bliss and my honor. The rest unfolds as it is.

APPENDIX B
ADDITIONAL EXERCISES
AND ACTIVITIES FOR
ALL CHAPTERS

CHAPTER 1 — UNREAL TO REAL: SNAPSHOTS OF MY STORY

Activities

1. Look at photographs of yourself throughout the years.
2. Write a letter to yourself as you see yourself in one or more of the photos.
3. Express your caring and describe how you are making your future better.
4. Mail this letter to yourself.

CHAPTER 2 — BEGINNING TO FREE YOURSELF

Learn different approaches to journaling and writing for healing: Read the works of Julia Cameron Janet Conner, Natalie Goldberg, Anne Lamott, and William Zinsser.

Chapter 3 — Early Warning Signs

Activities

1. Discover something in your home that is unsafe and repair it.
2. Discover places that nourish your heart or inspire your soul and spend time there regularly. For example, libraries, museums, places of worship.
3. Discover ways to care more for yourself: for example, organize your finances, get a medical checkup.

Chapter 4 — How Do I Begin Recovery?

Activities

1. Watch food-related movies
   - *Like Water for Chocolate* (2000)
   - *Babette's Feast* (1987)
   - *Chocolat* (2001)
   - *Cloudy with a Chance of Meatballs* (2009)
   - *Julie and Julia* (2009)
   - *Ratatouille* (2007)
2. Explore eating disorder recovery websites and blogs. Read stories

and comments from people working on their recovery.

CHAPTER 5 — BOUNDARIES: A CHALLENGE IN EARLY RECOVERY

Boundary Strengthening Activities
Money

1. Write every penny you spend in the course of a day for one week.
2. On day eight, look at where your money went. Include coins in parking meters. Include all check, cash, PayPal, and credit card purchases. Examine your patterns and choices. Total the money you spent. Think about your wishes and goals, how you live, and how you would like to live. Make a spending/saving budget for yourself based on what you value. Follow your budget for a week.
3. Journal about this experience and the challenges you discover. Explore where treats, necessities, impulse, and status issues might need different boundaries.

Saying No

Pay attention to how people say no in books, movies, stories, and political speeches. Journal about examples that could be helpful to you.

CHAPTER 6 — SECRETS

Activities
Recovery Journal Possibilities

1. Do an emotional check-in through-out your journal writing. Record your emotions on the page. Describe personal experiences that relate to what you are writing, including wishes and fantasies.
2. Describe risks or dangers you would encounter if you honored the issue. What might you gain if you honored the issue? What might you lose if you honored the issue?
3. In history or movies or the news or novels or memory, who addressed this issue badly or well? How can you learn from these examples?
4. Journal on living a life with no secrets.

Prompts For Healing And Growth Writings

- What values do I live by?
- Who am I trying to please?
- What are my secret desires?
- What are my cherished fantasies?
- What is my secret strength?
- What is my secret talent?
- What is my proudest moment?
- What is my most shameful moment?
- What could I do if I dared to try?

CHAPTER 7 — CHALLENGES TO EATING WELL

Activities

1. When you want to eat more than you know is right for you, consider all your senses. Have readily available something lovely for your eyes, ears, nose, and touch as well as taste. Give your other senses satisfaction.

2. When you are restricting, give your senses soothing and pleasure. Create a self-caring and kindness affirmation for yourself to allow you to receive needed nourishment.

3. Turn your scale into a work of art. Paint it or collage it. Make it use-

less as a scale and a pretty or fun
symbol of your growing freedom.

CHAPTER 8 — CONTEMPLATIONS ON EATING A MEAL

Activities

1. Explore how people of different cultures and religions practice respect for their food. Begin by exploring the heritage of your family.
2. Add mindful observation to your breathing exercise. Observe what is in your environment while doing your breathing exercise and take no action. Watch mindfully without regard for time and wait for: a shadow of a tree to reach a specific object; a cloud to pass a building; a bird to leave a branch; a wind chime to come to silence; twilight to turn to dark.

CHAPTER 9 — SPIRITUAL DEPTH

Activities

1. Explore the sacred ground of others — learn what sacred means to

you and to others. Is there a difference?

2. Give mindful attention to growing plants you see in your ordinary day.
3. Mindfully raise a plant in a pot on your windowsill, porch, or terrace.
4. Research the history and geography of land you know. Begin with your neighborhood.

CHAPTER 10 — THE GREAT TERROR

Activities

1. Create a writer's sketchbook. Choose a place. Stay there for forty-five minutes. Write continually what you hear and nothing else. After two hours or more, read what you wrote. Do this as often as you like, and especially when you are in the grip of fear.
2. Do a "kind question journal." For example, ask on paper, "What would nourish my heart and soul today?" Allow your wise self to respond. Schedule a time as soon as possible to follow your wisdom instructions.

Chapter 11 — Recovery Check-In

Complete these sentences and elaborate on them in your journal.

1. My new and more healthy and kind attitude toward food and my way of eating is _____.
2. I am creating a regular, gentle and kind way of giving my body strengthening exercise by _____.
3. With kindness and ease I am honoring my relationships with those I care for and who care for me by _____.
4. I am creating a regular check-in with myself to see if my attitude and my behaviors are in harmony with my health and recovery by _____.

Chapter 12 — Sex, Stalking, and Exploitation

1. Backtrack your past painful or dangerous sexual liaisons.
2. What could help you recognize a painful or dangerous sexual liaison?
3. What could help you protect yourself from a painful or dangerous liaison?
4. What makes a certain kind of sexual liaison dangerous for you? (Journal on your answers.)

5. Read *The Loser: Warning Signs You're Dating a Loser* by Joseph M. Carver, PhD.
6. If you feel threatened, visit *www .ndvh.org* or call:

 National Domestic Violence Hotline: 800-799-SAFE or 800-799-7233. Anonymous crisis intervention and referrals to resources, such as women's shelters. Available 24 hours every day.
7. Read the article "Domestic violence against women: Recognize patterns, seek help" at: *www.mayoclinic.com/ health/domestic-violence/WO00044*

CHAPTER 13 — FAMILY

Activities

1. Journal on what you see and feel while looking at family photographs and videos.
2. Use Google Maps to retrace and follow pathways of your past. Follow the arrow through the geography of your childhood.
3. Take a class in writing memoirs.

CHAPTER 14 — TRIGGERS AS TEACHERS: STAYING ON YOUR RECOVERY PATH

Activities

1. Make a list of activities that soothe and nourish you. Put them on separate pieces of paper in a box. Add to this box regularly. Every morning pick one at random and make that activity part of your day.
2. Read aloud and then speak to your reflection in the mirror, from memory, your chosen three affirmations.
3. Recovery work has a Rip Van Winkle aspect to it. In recovery you wake up, as if after a long sleep, to a different and more complex world. You may not have the knowledge or the credentials you need to pursue your dreams. Look for classes throughout your community. Look into the entrance requirements for a community college, state college, or university that will allow you to complete a degree or get an advanced degree.

■ ■ ■ ■

The internet offers many free opportunities for rich and in-depth learning. Bill Hogan's article, "How to Learn Just About Anything Online . . . For Free" in the *AARP Bulletin* print edition (January 1, 2010) lists over 22 sites that offer classes which include a syllabus, homework, exams, and audio or video lectures.

You can find the article online at: *www.aarp.org/personal-growth/life-long-learning/info-01-2010/learn_anything_online_for_free.html*

APPENDIX C
FACTS ABOUT EATING DISORDERS AND THE SEARCH FOR SOLUTIONS

This pamphlet was produced by the National Institute of Mental Health and is in the public domain.
NIH Publication No. 01-4901
First published in 2001;
updated August 06, 2002

Eating is controlled by many factors, including appetite, food availability, family, peers, and cultural practices, and attempts at voluntary control. Dieting to a body weight leaner than needed for health is highly promoted by current fashion trends, sales campaigns for special foods, and in some activities and professions. Eating disorders involve serious disturbances in eating behavior, such as extreme and unhealthy reduction of food intake or severe overeating, as well as feelings of distress or extreme concern about body shape or weight. Researchers are investigating how and why initially voluntary behaviors, such as eating smaller or larger amounts of food than usual, at some point move beyond control in some people and develop into an eating disorder.

Studies on the basic biology of appetite control and its alteration by prolonged overeating or starvation have uncovered enormous complexity, but in the long run have the potential to lead to new pharmacologic treatments for eating disorders.

Eating disorders are not due to a failure of will or behavior; rather, they are real, treatable medical illnesses in which certain maladaptive patterns of eating take on a life of their own. The main types of eating disorders are anorexia nervosa and bulimia nervosa.[1] A third type, binge-eating disorder, has been suggested but has not yet been approved as a formal psychiatric diagnosis.[2] Eating disorders frequently develop during adolescence or early adulthood, but some reports indicate their onset can occur during childhood or later in adulthood.[3]

Eating disorders frequently co-occur with other psychiatric disorders such as depression, substance abuse, and anxiety disorders.[1] In addition, people who suffer from eating disorders can experience a wide range of physical health complications, including serious heart conditions and kidney failure, which may lead to death. Recognition of eating disorders as real and treatable diseases, therefore, is critically important.

Females are much more likely than males to develop an eating disorder. Only an estimated 5 to 15 percent of people with anorexia or bulimia[4] and an estimated 35 percent of those with binge-eating disorder[5] are male.

ANOREXIA NERVOSA

An estimated 0.5 to 3.7 percent of females suffer from anorexia nervosa in their lifetime.[1] Symptoms of anorexia nervosa include:

- Resistance to maintaining body weight at or above a minimally normal weight for age and height
- Intense fear of gaining weight or becoming fat, even though underweight
- Disturbance in the way in which one's body weight or shape is experienced, undue influence of body weight or shape on self-evaluation, or denial of the seriousness of the current low body weight

- Infrequent or absent menstrual periods (in females who have reached puberty)

People with this disorder see themselves as overweight even though they are dangerously thin. The process of eating becomes an obsession. Unusual eating habits develop, such as avoiding food and meals, picking out a few foods and eating these in small quantities, or carefully weighing and portioning food. People with anorexia may repeatedly check their body weight, and many engage in other techniques to control their weight, such as intense and compulsive exercise, or purging by means of vomiting and abuse of laxatives, enemas, and diuretics. Girls with anorexia often experience a delayed onset of their first menstrual period.

The course and outcome of anorexia nervosa vary across individuals: some fully recover after a single episode; some have a fluctuating pattern of weight gain and relapse; and others experience a chronically deteriorating course of illness over many years. The mortality rate among people with anorexia has been estimated at 0.56 percent per year, or approximately 5.6 percent per decade, which is about 12 times higher than the annual death rate due to all causes of death among females ages 15–24 in the general population.[6] The most common causes of death are complications of the disorder, such as cardiac arrest or electrolyte imbalance, and suicide.

BULIMIA NERVOSA

An estimated 1.1 percent to 4.2 percent of females have bulimia nervosa in their lifetime.[1] Symptoms of bulimia nervosa include:

- Recurrent episodes of binge eating, characterized by eating an excessive amount of food within a discrete period of time and by a sense of lack of control over eating during the episode
- Recurrent inappropriate compensatory behavior in order to prevent weight gain, such as self-induced vomiting or misuse of laxatives, diuretics, enemas, or other medications (purging); fasting; or excessive exercise
- The binge eating and inappropriate compensatory behaviors both occur, on average, at least twice a week for 3 months
- Self-evaluation is unduly influenced by body shape and weight

Because purging or other compensatory

behavior follows the binge-eating episodes, people with bulimia usually weigh within the normal range for their age and height. However, like individuals with anorexia, they may fear gaining weight, desire to lose weight, and feel intensely dissatisfied with their bodies. People with bulimia often perform the behaviors in secrecy, feeling disgusted and ashamed when they binge, yet relieved once they purge.

BINGE-EATING DISORDER

Community surveys have estimated that between 2 percent and 5 percent of Americans experience binge-eating disorder in a 6-month period.[5,7] Symptoms of binge-eating disorder include:

- Recurrent episodes of binge eating, characterized by eating an excessive amount of food within a discrete period of time and by a sense of lack of control over eating during the episode
- The binge-eating episodes are associated with at least 3 of the following: eating much more rapidly than normal; eating until feeling uncomfortably full; eating large amounts of food when not feeling physically hungry; eating alone because of being embarrassed by how

much one is eating; feeling disgusted with oneself, depressed, or very guilty after overeating
- Marked distress about the binge-eating behavior
- The binge eating occurs, on average, at least 2 days a week for 6 months
- The binge eating is not associated with the regular use of inappropriate compensatory behaviors (e.g., purging, fasting, excessive exercise)

People with binge-eating disorder experience frequent episodes of out-of-control eating, with the same binge-eating symptoms as those with bulimia. The main difference is that individuals with binge-eating disorder do not purge their bodies of excess calories. Therefore, many with the disorder are overweight for their age and height. Feelings of self-disgust and shame associated with this illness can lead to bingeing again, creating a cycle of binge eating.

TREATMENT STRATEGIES

Eating disorders can be treated and a healthy weight restored. The sooner these disorders are diagnosed and treated, the better the outcomes are likely to be. Because of their complexity, eating disorders require a comprehensive treatment plan involving medical care and monitoring, psychosocial interventions, nutritional counseling and, when appropriate, medication management. At the time of diagnosis, the clinician must determine whether the person is in immediate danger and requires hospitalization.

Treatment of anorexia calls for a specific program that involves three main phases: (1) restoring weight lost to severe dieting and purging; (2) treating psychological disturbances such as distortion of body image, low self-esteem, and interpersonal conflicts; and (3) achieving long-term remission and rehabilitation, or full recovery. Early diagnosis and treatment increases the treatment success rate. Use of psychotropic medication in people with anorexia should be considered only after weight gain has been established. Certain selective serotonin reuptake inhibitors (SSRIs) have been shown to be helpful for weight maintenance and for resolving mood and anxiety symptoms associated with anorexia.

The acute management of severe weight loss is usually provided in an inpatient hospital setting, where feeding plans address the person's medical and nutritional needs. In some cases, intravenous feeding is recommended. Once malnutrition has been corrected and weight gain has begun, psychotherapy (often cognitive-behavioral or interpersonal psychotherapy) can help people with anorexia overcome low self-esteem and address distorted thought and behavior patterns. Families are sometimes included in the therapeutic process.

The primary goal of treatment for bulimia is to reduce or eliminate binge eating and purging behavior. To this end, nutritional rehabilitation, psychosocial intervention, and medication management strategies are often employed. Establishment of a pattern of regular, non-binge meals, improvement of attitudes related to the eating disorder, encouragement of healthy but not excessive exercise, and resolution of co-occurring conditions such as mood or anxiety disorders are among the specific aims of these strategies. Individual psychotherapy (especially cognitive-behavioral or interpersonal psychotherapy), group psychotherapy that uses a cognitive-behavioral approach, and family or marital therapy have been reported to be effective. Psychotropic medications, primarily antidepressants such as the selective serotonin reuptake inhibitors (SSRIs), have been found helpful for people with bulimia, particularly those with significant symptoms of depression or anxiety, or those who have not responded adequately to psychosocial treatment alone. These medications also may help prevent relapse. The treatment goals and strategies for binge-eating disorder are similar to those for bulimia, and studies are currently evaluating the effectiveness of various interventions.

People with eating disorders often do not recognize or admit that they are ill. As a result, they may strongly resist getting and staying in treatment. Family members or other trusted individuals can be helpful in ensuring that the person with an eating disorder receives needed care and rehabilitation. For some people, treatment may be long term.

RESEARCH FINDINGS AND DIRECTIONS

Research is contributing to advances in the understanding and treatment of eating disorders.

NIMH-funded scientists and others continue to investigate the effectiveness of psychosocial interventions, medications, and the combination of these treatments with the goal of improving outcomes for people with eating disorders.[8,9]

Research on interrupting the binge-eating cycle has shown that once a structured pattern of eating is established, the person experiences less hunger, less deprivation, and a reduction in negative feelings about food and eating. The two factors that increase the likelihood of bingeing hunger and negative feelings are reduced, which decreases the frequency of binges.[10]

Several family and twin studies are suggestive of a high irritability of anorexia and bulimia,[11,12] and researchers are searching for genes that confer susceptibility to these disorders.[13] Scientists suspect that multiple genes may interact with environmental and other factors to increase the risk of developing these illnesses. Identification of susceptibility genes will permit the development of improved treatments for eating disorders.

Other studies are investigating the neurobiology of emotional and social behavior relevant to eating disorders and the neuroscience of feeding behavior.

Scientists have learned that both appetite and energy expenditure are regulated by a highly complex network of nerve cells and molecular messengers called neuropeptides.[14,15] These and future discoveries will provide potential targets for the development of new pharmacologic treatments for eating disorders.

Further insight is likely to come from

studying the role of gonadal steroids.[16,17] Their relevance to eating disorders is suggested by the clear gender effect in the risk for these disorders, their emergence at puberty or soon after, and the increased risk for eating disorders among girls with early onset of menstruation.

FOR MORE INFORMATION

National Institute of Mental Health (NIMH)
Office of Communications and Public Liaison
Public Inquiries: (301) 443-4513
Web site: *www.nimh.nih.gov*

Harvard Eating Disorders Center
c/o Massachusetts General Hospital
15 Parkman Street
Boston, MA 02114
Phone: (617) 726-8470
Web site: *www.hedc.org*

National Association of Anorexia Nervosa and Associated Disorders
P.O. Box 7
Highland Park, IL 60035
Phone: (847) 831-3438
Web site: *www.anad.org*

National Eating Disorders Association
603 Stewart Street, Suite 803
Seattle, WA 98101
Phone: (206) 382-3587
Web site: *www.nationaleatingdisorders.org*

REFERENCES

1. American Psychiatric Association Work Group on Eating Disorders. Practice guideline for the treatment of patients with eating disorders (revision). *American Journal of Psychiatry,* 2000; 157(1 Suppl): 1–39.
2. American Psychiatric Association. *Diagnostic and Statistical Manual for Mental Disorders,* fourth edition (DSM-IV). Washington, DC: American Psychiatric Press, 1994.
3. Becker AE, Grinspoon SK, Klibanski A, Herzog DB. Eating disorders. *New England Journal of Medicine,* 1999; 340(14): 1092–8.
4. Andersen AE. Eating disorders in males. In: Brownell KD, Fairburn CG, eds. *Eating disorders and obesity: a comprehensive handbook.* New York: Guilford Press, 1995; 177–87.
5. Spitzer RL, Yanovski S, Wadden T, Wing R, Marcus MD, Stunkard A, Devlin M,

Mitchell J, Havein D, Horne RL. Binge eating disorder: its further validation in a multisite study. *International Journal of Eating Disorders,* 1993; 13(2): 137–53.

6. Sullivan PF. Mortality in anorexia nervosa. *American Journal of Psychiatry,* 1995; 152(7): 1073–4.

7. Bruce B, Agras WS. Binge eating in females: a population-based investigation. *International Journal of Eating Disorders,* 1992; 12: 365–73.

8. Agras WS. Pharmacotherapy of bulimia nervosa and binge eating disorder: longer-term outcomes. *Psychopharmacology Bulletin,* 1997; 33(3): 433–6.

9. Wilfley DE, Cohen LR. Psychological treatment of bulimia nervosa and binge eating disorder. *Psychopharmacology Bulletin,* 1997; 33(3): 437–54.

10. Apple RF, Agras WS. *Overcoming eating disorders. A cognitive-behavioral treatment for bulimia and binge-eating disorder.* San Antonio: Harcourt Brace & Company, 1997.

11. Strober M, Freeman R, Lampert C, Diamond J, Kaye W. Controlled family study of anorexia nervosa and bulimia nervosa: evidence of shared liability and transmission of partial syndromes. *Ameri-*

can *Journal of Psychiatry,* 2000; 157(3): 393–401.

12. Walters EE, Kendler KS. Anorexia nervosa and anorexic-like syndromes in a population-based female twin sample. *American Journal of Psychiatry,* 1995; 152(1): 64–71.

13. Kaye WH, Lilenfeld LR, Berrettini WH, Strober M, Devlin B, Klump KL, Goldman D, Bulik CM, Halmi KA, Fichter MM, Kaplan A, Woodside DB, Treasure J, Plotnicov KH, Pollice C, Rao R, McConaha CW. A search for susceptibility loci for anorexia nervosa: methods and sample description. *Biological Psychiatry,* 2000; 47(9): 794–803.

14. Frank GK, Kaye WH, Altemus M, Greeno CG. CSF oxytocin and vasopressin levels after recovery from bulimia nervosa and anorexia nervosa, bulimic subtype. *Biological Psychiatry,* 2000; 48(4): 315–8.

15. Elias CF, Kelly JF, Lee CE, Ahima RS, Drucker DJ, Saper CB, Elmquist JK. Chemical characterization of leptin-activated neurons in the rat brain. *Journal of Comparative Neurology,* 2000; 423(2): 261–81.

16. Devlin MJ, Walsh BT, Katz JL, Roose SP, Linkei DM, Wright L, Vande Wiele R,

Glassman AH. Hypothalamic-pituitary-gonadal function in anorexia nervosa and bulimia. *Psychiatry Research,* 1989; 28(1): 11–24.

17. Flanagan-Cato LM, King JF, Blechman JG, O'Brien MP. Estrogen reduces cholecystokinin-induced c-Fos expression in the rat brain. *Neuroendocrinology,* 1998; 67(6): 384–91.

APPENDIX D
RECOVERY JOURNAL
PROMPTS

GOALS:

1. Reach healthy body weight and optimum physical health. Journal prompts:
   - Nutrition
   - Sleep
   - Exercise
   - Hormonal balance
   - Teeth and gum restoration
   - Balanced electrolyte system
   - Regular medical check-ups

2. Heal psychological disturbances and wounds. Journal prompts:
   - Body image distortion
   - Continual harsh self-criticism
   - Recurrent conflict and problems in relationships
   - Bingeing
   - Starving

- Purging
- Excessive exercise
- Isolating

3. Stabilize long term recovery. Journal prompts:
   - Tolerate and understand feelings.
   - Healthy boundaries.
   - Boundaries of others.
   - End black and white thinking.
   - My genuine interests and goals.
   - How do I develop tools and skills to go for them?
   - Courage.
   - How do I remain present for what is?
   - Say no to what is not good for me.
   - Develop patience with others.
   - How do I learn to love?
   - How do I learn to accept love?
   - What is love?
   - What is dependence?
   - What is addictive need?
   - What is safety?
   - What structure do I need in my work, home, relationships?
   - Say yes to what is meaningful to you.

- How do I play?
- How can I avoid carrying a new secret?

Journal on any of these topics. You don't have to do them in order or all at once. Eating disorder recovery requires continual growth and development to cope with life challenges. Do an emotional check-in throughout your writing and put your feelings, wishes, and fantasies on the page.

APPENDIX E
HOW TO FIND MORE HELP

Find referrals from established and respected eating disorder professional associations, preferably those that require academic qualifications and eating disorder treatment experience for membership. These organizations can help you find mental health clinicians, physicians who have knowledge of eating disorders, nutritionists, and various in-patient and day treatment centers.

PROFESSIONAL ORGANIZATIONS
Academy for Eating Disorders (AED)
www.acadeatdis.org

American Anorexia and Bulimia
Association (AABA)
www.aabainc.org

International Association of Eating
Disorders Professionals (IAEDP)
www.iaedp.com

International Society for the Study of Dissociation
www.issd.org

International Society for Traumatic Stress Studies
www.istss.org

National Eating Disorders Association
www.nationaleatingdisorders.org

Sidran Foundation
www.sidran.org

Tip: You can contact any clinician who is a member of these organizations, briefly describe your situation and ask for a referral from any part of the world. Through the extensive networking available now through online member discussion lists, clinicians can request referrals and receive responses quickly (if resources are available in your location). This way you may get connected with clinicians who have some information about you and your situation and are prepared and willing to work with you.

FREE SUPPORTIVE RECOVERY MEETINGS
ANAD (National Association of Anorexia Nervosa and Associated Disorders)

354

Over 250 free support groups in the United States and in some foreign countries.
www.anad.org

OA Program of Recovery
Overeaters Anonymous offers a program of recovery from compulsive overeating using the Twelve Steps and Twelve Traditions of Alcoholics Anonymous.
www.oa.org/index.htm

Al-Anon/Alateen
Created over 50 years ago, Al-Anon and Alateen support and educate families and friends of alcoholics and help with creating and honoring personal boundaries — essential to eating disorder recovery.
www.al-anon.alateen.org/english.html

WEBSITES
Edreferral
Comprehensive online database of anorexia, bulimia, and other eating disorder treatment professionals worldwide.
edreferral.com

Something Fishy
A vast site of pro-recovery resources that's dedicated to raising awareness and providing support to people with eating disorders and their loved ones since 1995.
www.something-fishy.org

Eating Disorder Recovery for Women
Joanna Poppink's website and blog.
www.eatingdisorderrecovery.com

When you consider working with a professional:

1. Check them out.

    Most states have licensing boards you can access online. See if the clinician you are considering is in good standing. If you learn that the clinician has worked in different parts of the country or different countries check out their licensing in those places and if possible, find out why they moved.

2. Monitor performance.

    Recovery work involves stress and feelings of distress. At the same time, if you feel something might be wrong in your relationship with

your health care provider (physi-
cian, nutritionist, psychotherapist,
dentist, or physical therapist), please
get a second opinion from another
professional.
3. Mind Brain Stress Reduction
Course information:
   *www.umassmed.edu/Content.aspx
   ?id=4125 4&LinkIdentifier=id*
4. Mind Brain Stress Reduction —
Find a course worldwide:
   www.umassmed.edu/cfm/mbsr

RECOMMENDED READINGS
AND REFERENCES

FICTION

Mulock Craik, Dinah Maria. *The Little Lame Prince* (New York: Grosset & Dunlap, 1948).

Gardner, John. *Nickel Mountain* (New York: Alfred A. Knopf, 1973).

Hammett, Dashiell. *The Novels of Dashiell Hammett* (New York: Alfred A. Knopf, 1965). Includes: *Red Harvest, The Dain Curse, The Maltese Falcon, The Glass Key,* and *The Thin Man.*

James, P.D. All her mystery novels.

Jansson, Tove. *Moomintroll Series* (seven books), Avon Camelot, 1976.

Lewis, C. S. *The Chronicles of Narnia,* Scholastic, 1995. Caution: Read *The Magician's Nephew* as the fourth volume. Do not read it first, or you will lose the reader experience Lewis intended.

MacDonald, Ross. All of his mystery novels.

Milne, A.A., *The House at Pooh Corner,* Dell Publishing 1970 (first published 1928).

Rawling, J. K. *Harry Potter* (Books 1–7) (New York: Arthur A. Levine Books, 2009).

Sayers, Dorothy, all her mystery novels. Tip: read them in order of her writing.

SPIRITUALITY

Baynes, Wilhelm, *The I Ching.* Bollingen Series XIX, Princeton University Press, 17th printing 1980. (foreword by Carl Jung).

Blum, Ralph, H. *The Book of Runes,* St. Martin's Press, 1993.

Hanh, Thich Nhat, *Anger: Wisdom for Cooling the Flames,* Riverhead Trade, 2002.

Lelwica, Michelle M. *The Religion of Thinness,* Gurze Books, 2009.

MacHovec, Frank J. (trans.) *The Book of Tao,* The Peter Pauper Press, 1962.

Neidhardt, John (trans) *Black Elk Speaks: Being the Life Story of a Holy Man of the Oglala Sioux,* Lincoln: University of Nebraska, 1979 (original 1932).

Reps, Paul and Senzaki, Nyogen (compiled) *Zen Flesh Zen Bones, A Collection of Zen and Pre-Zen Writings,* Turtle Publishing, 1985.

Smart, Ninian & D. Hecht, Richard eds, *Sacred Texts of the World, a Universal Anthology,* Macmillan Publishers, Ltd., 1982.

Tolle, Eckhart, *The Power of Now: A Guide to Spiritual Enlightenment,* New World Library, 1999.

FAIRY TALES, MYTHS, AND LEGENDS

Bulfinch, Thomas, *Bulfinch's Mythology,* Spring Books, 1963.

Campbell, Joseph, *The Hero with a Thousand Faces,* Bollingen Series, Princeton, 1973.

Erdoes, Richard & Ortiz, Alfonso (selected and eds.) *American Indian Myths and Legends,* Panthelon Books, 1984.

Manheim, Ralph (trans) *Grimms' Tales for Young and Old, The Complete Stories,* Anchor Press/Doubleday, 1983.

Pinkola Estes, Clarissa, *Women Who Run with the Wolves,* Ballantine, 1996.

von Franz, Marie Louise, *The Interpretation of Fairy Tales,* Shambhala Publications, 1970.

von Franz, Marie Louise, *The Feminine in Fairy Tales,* Shambhala Publications, 1993.

Zipes, Jack, Ed., *Spells of Enchantment,* Penguin Books, 1992.

HUMAN DEVELOPMENT

Carver, Joseph, M. "The Loser: Warning Signs You're Dating a Loser," *www.drjoe carver.com/clients/49355/File/Identifying Losers.html*.

Erikson, Erik, *Childhood and Society,* New York, 1963 (original published in 1950).

Kohut, Heinz, *Restoration of the Self,* International Universities Press, 1977.

Kohut, Heinz, *How Does Psychoanalysis Cure?* University of Chicago Press, 1984.

Meloy, Reid, J., *Violent Attachments,* Jason Aronson Inc., 1992.

Meloy, Reid, J., (ed.) *The Psychology of Stalking,* Academic Press, 1998.

Miller, Alice, *The Drama of the Gifted Child,* Basic Books, 1981.

Newton, Ruth P., *The Attachment Connection,* New Harbinger Publications, 2008.

Rosenberg, Marshall, *Nonviolent Communication,* Puddledancer Press, 2003.

Schore, Alan, *Affect Regulation and the Origin of the Self,* Hillsdale, 1994.

Siegel, Daniel J. *The Developing Mind,* The Guilford Press, 1999.

Stern, D., *The Interpersonal World of the Infant: A View from Psychoanalysis and Developmental Psychology,* Basic Books, 1985.

Sroufe, L. Alan, Byron Egeland, Elizabeth A. Carolson, and W. Andrew Collins. *The Development of the Person,* The Guilford Press, 2005.

Walker, Barbara. *The Crone: Women of Age, Wisdom and Power.* HarperOne, 1988.

Woodman, Marion, *Addiction to Perfection,* Inner City Books, 1982.

Zinsser, William, *Writing to Learn,* Harper Paperbacks, 1993.

CONSCIOUSNESS

Bateson, Gregory, *Steps Toward an Ecology of the Mind,* Paladin, 1973.

Brande, Dorothea, *Wake Up and Live,* Simon & Schuster, 1980.

Cameron, Julia, *The Artist's Way,* Jeremy P. Tarcher/Putman, 2002.

Casey, Karen, *Change Your Mind and Your Life Will Follow,* Conari Press, 2005.

Conner, Janet, *Writing Down Your Soul,* Conari Press, 2008.

Covey, Stephen R. *The 7 Habits of Highly Effective People,* Fireside Book, 1989.

Damasio, Antonio, *The Feel of What Happens: Body and Emotion in the Making of Consciousness,* Harcourt Brace, 1999.

Edwards, Betty, *Drawing on the Right Side of the Brain,* Tarcher/ Putman, 1999.

Harvard Business Review, "On Work and Life Balance," Harvard Business School Press, 2000.

Kabat-Zinn, Jon, *Full Catastrophe Living,* Bantam Dell, 2005.

Musashi, Miyamoto, (Victor Harris trans) *The Book of Five Rings,* Overlook Press, 1974 (originally written, 1653).

Rico, Gabriele, *Writing Your Way Through Personal Crisis,* Tarcher/Putnam, 1991.

Watkins, Mary, *Invisible Guests,* Spring Publications, 2000.

Williams, Mark & Teasdale, John & Segal, Zindel & Kabat-Zinn, Jon, *The Mindful Way Through Depression,* The Guilford Press, 2007.

MEMOIR

Dillard, Annie, *The Writing Life,* Harper Perennial, 1990.

Field, Joanna, *A Life of One's Own,* J. P. Tarcher, 1981 (orig pub 1936).

Hornbacher, Marya, *Wasted: A Memoir of Anorexia and Bulimia,* New York: Harper-Flamingo, 1998.

Sacks, Oliver, *A Leg to Stand On,* A Touchstone Book published by Simon & Schuster, 1998.

Schweitzer, Albert (trans by Antje Bultmann Lemke) *Out of My Life and Thought,* Johns

Hopkins University Press in association
with the Albert Schweitzer Institute for
the Humanities (1933, 1949), 1998 edition (foreword by Jimmy Carter).

Wilkomirski, Binjamin (trans by Carol
Brown Janeway) *Fragments, Memories of a
Wartime Childhood.* Schocken Books,
1996.

Woolf, Virginia, *A Room of One's Own,* Harcourt Brace Jovanovich, 1929.

POETRY

Donne, John, *Collected Poems and Prose,*
Nonesuch, 1992 (written, 1624).

Eliot, T.S. *Four Quartets,* Harcourt, Brace
and Company, 1943.

AUDIOTAPES AND CDS

Hanh, Thich Nhat, *The Present Moment,*
Sounds True, 1993.

Kabat-Zinn, Jon, *Mindfulness for Beginners*
(Audiobook — June 1, 2006).

Kornfield, Jack, *The Inner Art of Meditation,*
Sounds True, 1993.

Kornfield, Jack, *Your Buddha Nature,* Sounds
True, 1997.

Woodman, Marion, *Dreams: Language of
the Soul,* Sounds True, 1990.

ABOUT THE AUTHOR

Joanna Poppink, MFT, is a licensed psychotherapist with more than twenty-five years of experience specializing in treating adults with eating disorders. She studied psychology at UCLA and the Saybrook Institute and received her master's degree from Antioch University. She lives in Los Angeles where, in addition to her practice, she finds time for improvisational theater, gardening, and playing on the beach with her family. She corresponds with women throughout the world via her website in her ongoing efforts to support eating disorder recovery.

Visit her at:.

www.eatingdisorderrecovery.com
Joanna@eatingdisorderrecovery.com
twitter.com/JoannaPoppink